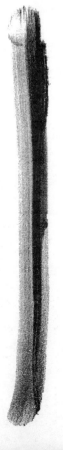

HE

To Burrumarra
and
other friends at Elcho Island.

*Cruel, Poor and Brutal
Nations* University of
Hawaii Press 1972
*Health in a Developing
Country* (with R M
Pulsford)
Jacaranda 1972
Medicine is the Law University
of Hawaii Press 1974
The Universe of the Warramirri
New South Wales
University Press 1993

UNSW
PRESS

ALERS
of
ARNHEM LAND

John Cawte

Photography by Douglass Baglin
Drawings by Billy Reid

Published by
UNIVERSITY OF
NEW SOUTH WALES PRESS
Sydney 2052 Australia
Telephone (02) 9398 8900
Facsimile (02) 9398 3408

National Library of Australia
Cataloguing-in-Publication entry:

Cawte, John
Healers of Arnhem Land.
ISBN 0 86840 351 2.

1. Yolngu (Australian people) —
Medicine. 2. Yolngu (Australian
people) — Health and hygiene.
3. Yolngu (Australian people) —
Folklore. 4. Aborigines, Australian
— Health and hygiene — Northern
Territory — Arnhem Land. I. Title.

306.0899915094295

The health centre at Galiwinku,
Elcho Island, Northern Territory will
receive 50 per cent of the
royalties from the sales of this book.

Design: Di Quick & Dana Lundmark
Editor: Carol Grabham
Managing Editor: Nada Madjar
Printer: McPhersons Printing
Publisher: Derelie Everly

CONTENTS

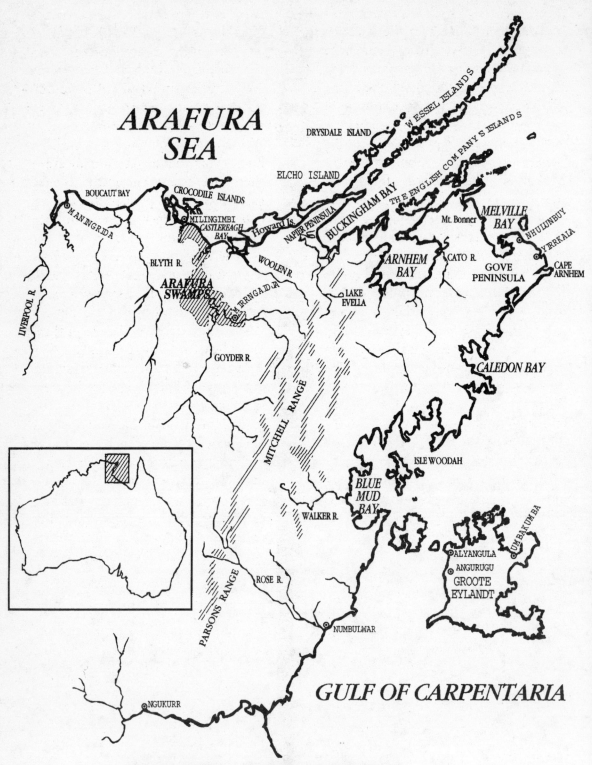

ARAFURA
SEA

DRYSDALE ISLAND

WESSEL ISLANDS

ELCHO ISLAND

THE ENGLISH COMPANY'S ISLANDS

BOUCAUT BAY

CROCODILE ISLANDS

MANINGRIDA

MILINGIMBI
CASTLEREAGH
BAY

Howard Is.

NAPIER PENINSULA

BUCKINGHAM BAY

Mt. Bonner

MELVILLE
BAY

NHULUNBUY

YIRRKALA

BLYTH R.

WOOLEN R.

ARNHEM
BAY

CATO R.

GOVE
PENINSULA

CAPE
ARNHEM

ARAFURA
SWAMPS

Mt IRRNGADJ R.

LAKE
EVELLA

LIVERPOOL R.

GOYDER R.

CALEDON BAY

MITCHELL RANGE

ISLE WOODAH

BLUE
MUD
BAY

WALKER R.

UMBAKUMBA

ALYANGULA

ANGURUGU

GROOTE
EYLANDT

PARSONS RANGE

ROSE R.

NUMBULWAR

GULF OF CARPENTARIA

NGUKURR

EAST ARNHEM
ABORIGINAL LAND

John Cawte is well known internationally as a pioneer in the study of variations in psychiatric phenomena according to culture. Commonly designated transcultural psychiatry, this field has been his lifelong interest and perhaps began with childhood experiences in Streaky Bay, South Australia, where some of his playmates were Aboriginal Australians. Even had he consciously chosen, given his English–Danish ancestry, Cawte could scarcely have picked a more interesting contrast between his cultural world and that of his childhood companions.

Over the past thirty-five years, John Cawte has published a steady stream of books and papers dealing with European–Aboriginal differences in forms and epidemiology of mental illnesses, notions about their cause and how they are managed. Perhaps his most important contribution has been his patient, year by year participation in the lives of these faraway peoples which has enabled his empathic entry into the thought worlds of at least a few of the major Aboriginal groups.

Cawte's in-depth knowledge and experience in medicine, psychiatry, anthropology and history permit him unusual bio-psycho-social perceptions. I remember the first time I heard Cawte lecture. He made the point that whereas long-distance European sea voyagers were plagued by scurvy, Indonesian colonisers of the Pacific never suffered scurvy even though their voyages were of equal duration. Long before the European discovery of the therapeutic and preventive value of limes and lemons, these intrepid seafarers carried tamarind pods which served the same preventive function. Cawte tossed tamarind pods to his audience to demonstrate how much more compact and convenient the tamarinds were than cargoes of fresh limes.

This present collection deals with the Yolngu of Arnhem Land in the Northern Territory, one of some 500 cultural groups comprising the original settlers. Cawte emphasizes that Aboriginal groups should not all be lumped together as they usually are— there are many culturally diverse groups which are perhaps as different one from the other as are Irish from Italian Europeans.

These writings represent a distinct departure from Cawte's earlier publications. He modestly refers to them as 'stories', but they certainly are unusual stories. Indeed it is difficult to fit them into any known category. Perhaps they are unique to John Cawte! These writings escape the purely literary or scientific but present actuality on the ground in Arnhem Land and, in so doing, they communicate the pervasive anxiety of a people caught up in sorcery, social threat and impending cultural obliteration. Cawte evokes a kind of verbal magic, conjuring multidimensional images by juxtaposing Yolngu and European forms of consciousness.

Most of the stories are based on detailed descriptions of Yolngu life: case histories of illness or misfortune; odd biographical incidents; or unusual self-revelations. These incidents are intertwined with subjective interpretations in both scientific and mythic terms. There are medical descriptions of leprosy and of the causative organism side by side with Yolngu conviction that the disease is the result of 'pay-back' or magical retaliation for misdeeds against a neighbouring clan. There are biological details of the remarkable box jellyfish or sea wasp that delivers paralysis and death through tiny grenades that explode under the victim's skin. My favourite story deals with the trade in the sea cucumbers or sea-ginseng which was a prized medicament to bolster the sexual appetites of jaded Chinese aristocrats. Macassans from Celebes brought home the sea-ginseng they had harvested and prepared; traders brought their silver from mainland China. This trade had developed about the time of Columbus and was first described for Westerners in the delightful journals of English naviga- tor Matthew Flinders (1774–1814). Cawte transcribes several pages for us here. Incidentally, I made the discovery that if you read these stories very carefully, you will even find flashes of English poetry—William Wordsworth, John Donne and Edward Fitzgerald—which illuminate the text from odd and unexpected angles.

In all of these stories and indeed the entire corpus of John Cawte's writing lies a pervasive, but somehow understated, sense of humanism. I recently came upon a passage written by Edward John Eyre (1815–1901) which perhaps best expresses Cawte's implicit humanism. It was Eyre of course who, a century ago and accom- panied by Wylie, his loyal Aboriginal guide, made the harrowing thousand- mile trek across the burning and waterless coast of the Great Aus- tralian Bight. They set out on their famous trek from Fowler's Bay, on that same coast where John Cawte was raised. Eyre wrote: 'It is a lamentable thing to think that the progress and prosperity of one race should conduce to the downfall and decay of another'.

Healers of Arnhem Land sounds a more positive note than the one struck by Edward John Eyre. The pulse of the Yolngu, felt by this observer, suggests that they are rallying, whatever their hardships and adversities.

Prof. Raymond Prince MD
Former Editor of *Transcultural Psychiatric Research Review*
Division of Social and Transcultural Psychiatry
McGill University
Montreal Canada

PREFACE

The 'top end' of Australia that lies to the east of Darwin is home to many culturally distinctive clans known collectively as the Yolngu of northeast Arnhem Land. For two decades between 1970 and 1990 during summer vacations, I made annual visits to the Yolngu, staying at the town of Galiwin'ku on Elcho Island. My motive was to offer support from my two medical specialities, for casualties of rapid cultural change and of exotic diseases, as described in this book.

The island people responded warmly to the interest that I took in their ways of healing and my role as medical adviser extended to that of a friend to the Yolngu and clan brother to David Burrumarra, leader of the Warramirri. The clans taught the benefit of the modern doctor immersing himself in the thinking of the people, gaining empathy with their motivations rather than simply proffering good advice.

The desire of the clan leaders that their traditional knowledge should not be lost led them to approach me with the request to record some of their songs and art in a book, subsequently published in 1993 as *The Universe of the Warramirri*. Now this book, *Healers of Arnhem Land*, summarises my many exchanges with members of the other Yolngu clans who invited this doctor into their midst. The clan leaders also arranged for healing scenes to be enacted for the camera and numerous photographs from the film appear in this book. The leader of the Galpu clan at that time, Monyu, who is mentioned in chapter 9, organised many of these enactments.

As this book is directed to readers of English, I have excluded dialect as far as possible. Dialect enabled my preceding book to cover more of Warramirri poetry, art and their world view generally. By contrast, this book is directed to a wider public— one that is interested in the fundamental issues of traditional healing as well as in the adversities now encountered by the indigenous people. A brief word list is provided for reference.

The people have happily retained their names in the local languages, not translating them to English as occurred with the American Indians. To preserve anonymity, however, I have translated individual names into English in a form that does not correspond with the meaning of the original. The exception to this convention is in chapter 6 where my colleague, Dr John Hargrave, chose to fabricate Yolngu names which sound more like the original.

The Yolngu of Arnhem Land endured this scorching earth for millennia. They survived it by living in mobile clans, not in settled communities. The endeavour to settle, at their level of technology, was catastrophic. It inflicted upon them crises of health and well-being that tend to overwhelm them today.

This book breaks new ground. It is one doctor's contribution to the well-being of a group of Yolngu clans in Arnhem Land, deriving from his attempt to span the gulf between white and black cultures. During a lifetime of medical care of Aborigines, I developed the view that sound medicine is not enough. If suffering individuals are to be reached, the doctor should try to grasp the patient's language, religion and basic beliefs. Unless the cultural gulf is narrowed in this way, there will be limited compliance with care.

Healers of Arnhem Land is not meant to invoke guilt in white or black readers. Information and tolerance are its goals. True, it deals with the anxiety and idioms of distress prevalent in Arnhem Land, but it seeks to present them as intriguing mysteries, threats and challenges, to be tackled by black and white. The people of Elcho Island are doing this, in my view.

Clearly this modest volume is not intended as an overview of tropical pathology. The great texts properly expound the infectious and parasitic features of exotic diseases. What is needed is a reminder of the person behind the disease and of that person's distinctive cultural interpretation. Obviously the cultural perspectives will be different in each community not yet overtaken by Western thought. In the vernacular of anthropologists, this book offers the 'emic' view—from within—of what is presented predominantly as an 'etic' discipline—seen from without.

In pursuit of this emic or inner view, we shall hearken to the voices of the patients in our chosen community. How do those affected by endemic diseases view their afflictions? What is their responsive repertoire? How may their world view affect their compliance with the regimens prescribed by Western medicine to combat the diseases?

Why call the conditions which they endured 'exotic diseases'? I do not use the term 'exotic' in its sense of the colourful or picturesque. 'Exotic disease' should make that clear. The habitat is exotic, in the sense of foreign, unusual, distinctively strange. It would be hard to find a more exotic place than the islands of the South Arafura Sea, some ten or eleven degrees below the equator, on the meridian of Irian Jaya. It is part of Australia, though some of the inhabitants scarcely know it. To them it is the land of the Yolngu clans of northeast Arnhem Land.

I call the diseases exotic because the term tropical or geographical is not suitable. Tropical medicine might be more accurately described as medicine in the tropics. Physicians who practise in the temperate zones, however, are encountering these problems with growing frequency as people travel more on business and for pleasure. Many of these conditions are rare in the temperate zones only because of the improved nutrition, housing and sanitation there.

The exhaustive tomes of tropical medicine rarely focus on traditional medicine. The failure of rapprochement between modern and traditional medicine in Papua New Guinea was analysed in 1972 in *Health in a Developing Country*, by R L Pulsford and myself. If we turn to the individuals who become sick among the Yolngu clans of Arnhem Land, the crucial question focuses again on the rapprochement of modern and traditional medicine. How can such a rapprochement be achieved? How may it help the sufferer, as well as the provider of health care? The Yolngu have some answers for us in this critical matter.

The present settlement at Galiwin'ku, on Elcho Island in Arnhem Land, owes much to its founder, Harold Shepherdson. I was fortunate to enjoy the support and hospitality of Harold and his wife Ella over many years and my deep appreciation goes to them.

Elcho Islanders gave consistent help during my many visits. When I had finalised this manuscript, with the aim that it would prove medically helpful, not only to this community but to others and to Australians at large, I sent it to a small but representative committee for approval. I would like to thank especially Oscar Datjarranga (Chairman of Council), Hilton Jones R.N. (Health Centre), Stephanie Yirkaniwuy (Senior Health Worker), George Danygambul (Director of Outlying Communities) and Carol Ward (Director of Nursing/ Community Care, Nhulunbuy).

Thanks are due to all the healers who enacted the healing sequences presented as photographs in this book. The clan leaders who arranged the demonstrations correspond closely with the group that approved my work for *The Universe of the Warramirri* (as listed in the table). My frequent medical companion was Dr H.B. (Don) Eastwell, who joined me from both Darwin and Brisbane. Don's experience of transcultural psychiatry was invaluable for me in my work.

Field experience has taught me that a doctor is the wrong person for the camera. Posing subjects infallibly destroys the link. Most (not all) of the colour photographs were taken by my friend Douglass Baglin. I thank him for his help on many trips to Galiwin'ku, where he was on friendly terms with the Yolngu. Unlike myself he could retire unobtrusively behind the camera, taking plenty of shots. The people trusted him.

Dr John Hargrave, formerly Medical Superintendent of East Arm Leprosarium near Darwin and writer on leprosy, frequently visited Elcho Island over Christmas. He and I shared some ten successive Christmas dinners as guests of the Shepherdsons; just the four of us, as the Shepherdsons had no family. Dr Hargrave provided for this volume the reflections of one of his patients, designed to indicate the impact of Hansen's disease on lifestyle.

The sick bay was attended by two hard-worked registered nurses (their numbers grew as the years passed). They tackled a wide range of problems of a kind never seen during their training. The most recent nurse in this distinguished line is Hilton Jones, who helped with this manuscript. My tribute to them is made in chapters 13 and 14.

The sick bay also provides an oasis for health workers from the population. I especially thank Yirkaniwuy, the current Senior Health Worker, and Djoimi. Many of them became competent performers in this setting.

The illustrator for *The Aboriginal Health Worker* during much of my editorship of the quarterly was a Kamilaroi artist from Bourke called Billy Reid. We are close friends, and he often came with me on field trips. Some of his illustrations are reproduced in this book. How he afflicted me with a nasty coral laceration is told in chapter 13 with his self-portrait.

During the time that I visited Elcho Island, the Council and the Church Missionary Society at Angurugu on Groote Eylandt invited me to study a paragon of exotic diseases, a nameless disorder of the brain that occurred

ACKNOWLEDGEMENTS

only in their vicinity. Eventually my colleagues and I identified the disorder as Joseph-Machado disease, a rare condition peculiar to the Portuguese. It is called 'the stumbling disease' among Azorean-Portuguese. How did it arrive in Australia? Angurugu was host to several exemplary researchers, including the ethnobotanist Dulcie Levitt, working to produce the study that is the best account of ethnobotany for any locality. Ms Levitt permitted me to furnish the extract on the traditional healing of wounds.

A regular port of call, coming and going, was Nhulunbuy and its branch of the Northern Territory Department of Health. I was always welcomed at Gove airport and lodged overnight at the quarters of the district hospital. Evenings were spent with the district medical officers, sharing views and concerns. There was often much more. Dr Stan Linco reliably took me on his fishing excursions to Melville Bay shoreline, where crocodiles lurked. Dr Henning Madsen and his wife Maria put on a Danish meal while we discussed everything from Copenhagen to Arnhem Land. I also thank other Regional Directors of Health, including John Quinn, Tom Gavranic, Max Chalmers, Ernie Lindfield and Margaret Sheridan. Sister Carol Ward, of Community Health Services, was always helpful.

The next morning a light plane would take me on the bumpy ride to the scorching earth at Elcho Island where my friends and helpers were expecting me. I must thank the successive chairmen of the Town Council, the councillors, and the clan leaders, too many to name here. Especially I thank George Danygambul, now Director of Outstation Services, for his encouragement for my work.

Communications with Canberra were also lively. I was regularly asked to discuss casualties of change at the Commonwealth Health Department and the Department of Aboriginal Affairs (as they were then called). Several of their senior officers, such as Denis Stanbury, Don O'Rourke and Bill Wilson, always wanted to know more of the idiom of distress in Arnhem Land.

Colleagues in the medical school at the University of New South Wales were invaluable in their support for my activities. I offer my thanks in particular to Professor L B Brown, Head of Psychology, Professor L G Kiloh, Head of Psychiatry; Professor Darty Glover, Dean of the Faculty of Medicine; Professor Bruce Warren, Head of Pathology at Prince Henry Hospital. This hospital kindly houses in cabinets in the administration building my precious set of artefacts used by traditional doctors, the only museum of its kind.

The United States of America showed high interest in my avocation. The following pages were first drafted at the Center for Advanced Study in the Behavioral Sciences at Stanford, California. I am grateful to the Center for their invitation to me for this purpose. Louis A Allen, of Palo Alto, California, is president of the international consulting firm of Louis A Allen Associates, Inc, and author of a number of books in the management field. He became a foremost collector of Arnhem Land art. Mr Allen remains a valuable helper to me in the publication of medical material overseas. Everyone at the University of New South Wales Press particularly Derelie Everly, Di Quick, and Nada Madjar deserve special thanks for their constant encouragement.

THE ROLL OF CLAN LEADERS WHO AGREED

17 February 1976 meeting

Burrumarra	Chairman	Mala (Clan) Leader	Warramirri
Djorrpum		Mala (Clan) Leader	Guy-yula Djambarrpuyngu
Djupandawuy		Mala (Clan) Leader	Gupapuynu Biunkidi
Matjuwi		Mala (Clan) Leader	Gomatj
Nyibayna		Mala (Clan) Leader	Dhalwanu
Barrnyunyur		Mala (Clan) Leader	Dhalwanu
Dayburryun (1)		Mala (Clan) Leader	Dadiwuy
Muwarra		Mala (Clan) Leader	Dadiwuy
Monyu		Mala (Clan) Leader	Galpu
Liwukan		Mala (Clan) Leader	Warramirri

6 May 1976 meeting

Burrumarra	Chairman	Mala (Clan) Leader	Warramirri
Nulpurray		Mala (Clan) Leader	Warramirri
Matjuwi		Mala (Clan) Leader	Gomatj
Liwukan		Mala (Clan) Leader	Warramirri
Buthiman		Mala (Clan) Leader	Wangurri
Wili Walalipa		Mala (Clan) Leader	Gulamala
Banbaitjun		Mala (Clan) Leader	Liyagawumirr Chairman
Djurrkuwidi		Mala (Clan) Leader	Guy-yula Djambarrpuyngu
Djorrpum		Mala (Clan) Leader	Guy-yula Djambarrpuyngu
Dayburryun (1)		Mala (Clan) Leader	Dadiwuy
Dayburryun (2)		Mala (Clan) Leader	Liyagawumirr
Djati		Mala (Clan) Leader	Gomatj
Barripan		Mala (Clan) Leader	Gulpa

17 May 1976 meeting

Burrumarra	Chairman	Mala (Clan) Leader	Warramirri
Badaitja		Mala (Clan) Leader	Wangurri
Dayburryun (2)		Mala (Clan) Leader	Liyagawumirr
Djorrpum		Mala (Clan) Leader	Guy-yula Djambarrpuyngu
Mandjuwi		Mala (Clan) Leader	Galpu
Muwarra		Mala (Clan) Leader	Dadiwuy
Lalabarri (1)		Mala (Clan) Leader	Dhalwanu
Burrminy (1)		Mala (Clan) Leader	Dhurrili Djambarrpuyngu
Gunbuku (1)		Mala (Clan) Leader	Guy-yula Djambarrpuyngu
Bulambi (2)		Mala (Clan) Leader	Dhalwanu

Of ARNH

PULSE

Medical examination by the sense o
radial artery at the wrist to registe
Are the beats rapid or slow? Strong o
Much is learned from this simple tec
face. The very act of taking the puls
doctor's part to help an anxious perso
lying sentiments in society or politic
rather than by open enquiry. The socia
like the pulse felt by the doctor from

Pulse seems the right term for the vitality, or throb of life, in Galiwin'ku, a new Aboriginal town in Arnhem Land. Arnhem Land is a broad expanse of Northern Australia, largely a barren plateau, occupied by a group of distinctive indigenous clans known as the Yolngu. They have maintained more of their traditional culture than has occurred elsewhere across the Australian subcontinent. For this reason, the area is immensely interesting to science and medicine.

The term Yolngu (roughly pronounced 'Jung who') connotes an Aboriginal person in all dialects of the region. The term Balanda is likewise applied to white people; it derives from 'Hollander', the word originally used to describe the Europeans coming to South-East Asia. The region was named after the Dutch ship *Arnhem*, which explored the Australian coastline in 1623 on a voyage from the Dutch East Indies.[1]

ouch is called palpation. Doctors and nurses palpate the
he successive beats of the heart. How does the wall feel?
veak? Regular or irregular? Of high pressure or low?
nique. Patients sense this; they scrutinise the doctor's
indicates both the expertise and the intent on the
Pulse is also used in a metaphorical way, for the under-
especially as discoverable by tact or skill in perception
nd economic pulse of the state tells much, rather
vatient's wrist.

EM LAND

Galiwin'ku began as recently as 1942, during World War II, when the Japanese Imperial Air Force was bombing towns along the northern coastline. One of the targets was Milingimbi mission[2] in the Crocodile Islands. The Milingimbi airstrip was being used by the RAAF for its Beaufort squadron. Beaufighters were a comparatively quiet aircraft, known for that reason as 'silent death' in the RAAF. Flying low, they could inter-cept Japanese aircraft and put them to flight. In these defensive sorties the RAAF was helped by the radar station hidden on Marchinbar,[3] the most northerly of the Wessel Islands that extend into the Arafura Sea.

Milingimbi, being an RAAF base, became the target of repeated Japanese air raids. In one attack, a missionary and several children were killed while taking shelter in a trench. It looked as though the raids would become more fierce and frequent, as they had in Darwin. The future was anxiously discussed at the Mission. Harold Shepherdson, a young missionary from Adelaide with skills in saw-milling and building, volunteered to take a Yolngu group from the Mission across the vast Castlereagh Bight to establish a new centre on Elcho Island to the east. Hopefully it would be unobserved by the enemy. The vicinity also offered good timber (native oaks) for house-building. Several senior Yolngu at Milingimbi undertook to help him.[4]

Harold Shepherdson's aim was never to establish a large community on

Elcho Island. One of his special gifts made him an ideal founder—his enthusiasm for flying. He even built a Heath Parasol for himself, later crashing it on Groote Eylandt. He survived. In these fragile aircraft, he could visit outlying communities, where people were living a mobile life in groups of up to 60. He told me that he flew to their homelands to keep them supplied with tobacco. Otherwise, without steady supplies of this addicting substance, most of the remote groups would have moved to the supply point at Galiwin'ku. He wanted to forestall this influx. He conducted Christian services on his visits, with the help of a tape recorder.[5]

When I first visited Galiwin'ku it was small. About 350 Yolngu were there, deriving from a dozen or more regional clans. There was a team of missionaries, hard at work teaching basic trades. I saw a row of tin sheds, comprising sawmill, carpentry workshop, motor repairs, power supply and store. A little church stood apart at the top of the rise. Fruit trees, such as mangoes and bananas, were growing round about. The people had been deterred from their camp habit of cutting down native trees, by order of the missionary. It was a shady place to live. Fishing, forest plantation and gardens were all being fostered. The forest was planted with native pines (*callitris*), a tree that is resistant to termites, indefatigable predators of other woods used for building. So the sawmill was set up, with men who could run it under training.

Between 1970 and 1990 I visited Elcho Island regularly as a medical doctor experienced in psychiatry and anthropology.

Cultural psychiatry is the name of the academic discipline to which I devoted much of my professional lifetime. Transcultural and cross-cultural psychiatry are alternative names for the discipline. I was inevitably directed to it by my life of association with Aborigines.[6]

Psychiatrists are essentially trained to make a relationship with the suffering individual. They must first try to achieve rapport and trust. Then they should review the remedial pattern most likely to be of help—be it in the fields of biology, psychology, interpersonal relations or social intervention. Which stress—in which of these four stressful universes—can the psychiatrist help to reduce? This may be a very complex prescription; it applies to Yolngu as much as to Balanda.

Is this an insoluble quandary? If anything, suffering seems greater among the Yolngu. Vital strivings are more likely to be blocked for them by the collapse of their culture today. Alexander Leighton emphasized that disintegrated social conditions were an important source of mental illness. A disintegrated community, Leighton deduced, will experience associated phenomena, such as a recent history of disaster; widespread ill-health; extensive poverty; confusion occasioned by the coexistence of two or more cultures that have no ordered relationship; widespread secularisation with an absence of religious sentiments; extensive in-or-out migration; and recent widespread cultural (for example, technological) change.[6]

My personal undertaking at this time in the early 1970s was to inaugurate a modest quarterly journal, *The Aboriginal Health Worker*. It was phrased in simple English and it tried to be accurate and practical. The government agreed to circulate it free of charge to the new professional helpers from the indigenous communities around Australia. Readers of the journal were invited to share their experiences and to think of themselves as founders of a new profession, crucial to their people. Aboriginal contributors to the journal were sought first and foremost.

During the thirteen years that I produced this homely journal, I chose not to focus unduly on traditional ways of healing. Had this been done, it would certainly have come under attack as an official policy; this would have threatened the modest funding that made the journal possible. Despite this, in my own practice I felt bound to explore the ideas of my patients about the source and management of their trouble. Failure to do this would have left the job half done. What the patient believes is a deciding factor in the outcome, and the response to treatment offered by somebody beyond the culture.

An elder who lives in Arnhem Land, and who has long been my friend, confided to me that the health programs for his people won't work: there are too many 'devil devils' out there, in the swamps and the scrub. This elder is so convinced of the satanic power of evil spirits to deliver illness and death that I would not argue with him. It has been his heritage all his life.

In Australian pidgin, devil devil, as the reduplicative form of devil, indicates intensity and magnitude. In tribal belief, devil devil is an evil spirit, a manifestation of evil, or evil itself. If you hear a tribesman talking about 'devil devil business', he is probably referring to a severe and mysterious sickness, for which singing and rituals must be perfused into the prostrate body to cleanse it.

Some doctors—especially those who practise in cities—are forced to work too fast. A few are slower. Decades of unhurried but more intimate exchange with Aboriginal patients in the outback lead me to agree that most of them do in fact inhabit a devil devil land. We don't have to employ the reduplication of pidgin to characterise their adversities. But identify these devil devils we must, otherwise health services will fail to respond to them.

The first may be called, in modern terms, adverse human ecology. These settlement dwellers live in an ecology that may act as foe more than as friend. This is conspicuously true of camp populations into which the clans clustered within living memory, as authorities tried to merge clans into communities. Few if any of these camps ever possessed the resources required for health.

Adverse human ecology is the first, and chief, phalanx in this devil devil land. City dwellers are often fascinated by the ambiguous ecology of Australia in its remoter regions. In these pages the central figures indicate customary Aboriginal responses to exotic hazards, such as the hookworm infestation of camps, deadly jellyfish, venomous snakes, toxic native foods, virulent fish and the invisible army of micro-organisms. These actors in our dramas offer us warnings of the exotic diseases.

The second devil devil of this beleaguered land is more subtle: so subtle, indeed, that many observers do not see it at all. It may be called the projective thinking of the tribes. This includes the curses and pay-back when people in pain blame it on the ill-will of enemies. Enemies need not be outsiders—they may be neighbours in the same camp. Their devil devil has been sent on a sinister errand by someone paying back a grudge, long inflamed and festered over.

Health providers may be unaware of these secrets. There is an inherent paranoia about curses and pay-back that keeps them secret from non-participants. These attitudes are undergoing revision from education, but they will not dissipate overnight. They may be re-invoked during the stress of maladies and misfortunes. These patterns are identified in the dramas portrayed. Curses and pay-back can pounce like a vicious dingo. Wounds quickly grow inflamed in this scorching miasma.

Which devil devil of this miasma is more hazardous? It depends where we look. In the dramas privileged to us, the dominant antagonist of the race is probably not the malice expected from jealous fellow tribesmen, cultivating hatred in their hearts. Rather, it is the unforgiving world around. If the sufferers then seek solace in alcohol, this devil devil grows to monstrosity. It looms over all, spitting distress and destruction. This is a scorching earth!

Scenes of healing

It is difficult to study healers in Arnhem Land—they do not run a clinic, or put up a brass plate! At Galiwin'ku, their identity was shielded. This happened not only because they prefer to practise in private. Out of deference to the health centre, they conducted healing ceremonies elsewhere, by lonely beaches and billabongs. I had seen little of it, despite all the talk. The leader of the Warramirri clan, Burrumarra, felt strongly that clan secrets should go into a book, rather than be hidden in the forest or underground. There was concern that traditional ways would be lost. The

leaders were all the more keen because they saw that in my earlier volume dealing with traditional healing among the tribes of Australia, every tribal region seemed to be represented except Arnhem Land.[7] Even if they could not read the words, the photographs fascinated them. So when the clan leaders offered to show me some of their ceremonies out in the bush, I was enthralled and full of questions. What is the drill for snakebite? Toothache? Constant coughing? Weariness?

The clan leaders were eager to cooperate, rounding up some 50 to 60 Yolngu to demonstrate. They and the actors were happy to have it filmed.[8] By and large it was the Galpu clan that came to the fore, but all of the volunteers performed with elan. They were not just play-acting; they were expressing conviction in their old ceremonies.

Cameraman Douglass Baglin and I recently discussed these photographs of scenes of healing, enacted for me in the early 1970s by Yolngu helpers and friends. It was our view that the best people to comment upon these photographs are those Yolngu who enacted them. I sent colour copies of several traditional healing scenes to the senior health worker at Galiwin'ku. I asked if she would consult with the chairman of the Council to decide if the original actors might be approached and furnish information on the kinds of scenes they portrayed. To the time of writing, no response has been received.

With regard to the photographs in this chapter, I have merely supplied an identifying caption, together with a brief comment. An exception is the first of the series of plates, bearing the caption 'Marngitj (medicine man) in the Arafura Swamps'. I have extended my commentary enough for the reader to appreciate some nuances of the situation in its broad ramifications. This has not been done for the remainder of the photographs. I could have provided this but Mr Baglin and I feel that this is the prerogative of the Yolngu concerned, should they wish to expand on the knowledge they were generous enough to share with us.

The scenes that we were privileged to witness took place out in the bush, away from the settlement, away from the white company, away from the sick bay. Don't discount them for that! In my view, they are still archetypes of Arnhem Land, part of its subconscious; a power in its pulse.

1 The skipper of the *Arnhem* and nine of his men had been killed by 'savages' of New Guinea with whom they tried to parley. Carstenz, skipper of the companion yacht *Pera*, sailed south to Cape York Peninsula, as the region is now called.

Carstenz's discoveries rendered his journal a joyless one for his commercial masters. He reported, 'We have not seen one fruit-bearing tree, nor anything men can make use of . . . In our judgement this is the most arid and barren region that could be found anywhere on earth. The inhabitants, too, are the most wretched and the poorest creatures that I have ever seen'. From beings of such a level it was hardly to be expected that much information could be gleaned; nor could the Dutch study individuals at leisure, for when they tried to capture specimens, these people were strangely reluctant to be rescued from their barren home! The reader should turn to a historian for a full account, for example, Beaglehole J C (1966) *The Exploration of the Pacific* (3rd edn) Stanford University Press.

2 American W Lloyd Warner lodged at this mission to compile the revealing study *A Black Civilisation* (1937). The Yolngu first gained widespread attention in this study as the 'Murngin'. Warner may not have endured fieldwork under conditions as rigorous as some readers imagine from his book. He lodged at the Methodist mission on Milingimbi Island, where Sister Jessie Smith, in charge of the health clinic, attended to his laundry and baked his daily bread. Jessie did the same for me, decades later.

3 This radar station (or Radio Direction Finding, RDF, as it was then known) was successfully camouflaged from the Japanese through the help of a Wessel Island man, Djingalul. I looked after Djingalul in his final years at Galiwin'ku. He was the last of the Wessel Islanders, old, frail and tired of life. It was my custom to enquire into the English meaning of vernacular names. To my surprise, Djingalul informed me that his name had no meaning in his own tongue—it was his attempt to say the English word 'jungle'! He was named after the mangrove jungle of his homeland, but this name was never used. He tried to translate it for the RAAF crew.

4 One of the volunteers was the boat captain, Wili Walalipa, a Yolngu of part-Indonesian (Macassan) descent. Wili later helped me, after my arrival, as I shall tell.

5 An intimate account of Shepherdson's work has been preserved in an illustrated book by Ella Shepherdson, *Half a Century in Arnhem Land*, compiled and published in 1981 by Ella and Harold Shepherdson, One Tree Hill, South Australia.

6 There was no training in this field in Australia. Fortunately, I was able to gain exposure to some of the leading authorities in the field in the USA during my formative professional years. In the 1950s, I was able to sit in with the Canadian transcultural psychiatrist Alexander H Leighton at Harvard University, and I tapped the minds of others eminent in this field, including Margaret Mead, Erich Fromm and Clyde Kluckhohn. I even shared an appointment in an establishment in Washington DC of the US Navy with Thomas S Szasz who titled his popular 1961 book *The Myth of Mental Illness*. My attachment to the same company was purely coincidental. My position about mental illness never became as extreme as Tommy's. Mental illness is no myth!

7 Cawte J (1974) *Medicine is the Law: Studies in Psychiatric Anthropology of Australian Tribal Societies* The University Press of Hawaii.

8 The half-hour film from which the photographs in this book are taken is entitled *Aboriginal Healing in Arnhem Land*. This film has attracted close medical interest around the world—even in the former Soviet Union.

WITH HIM intent to

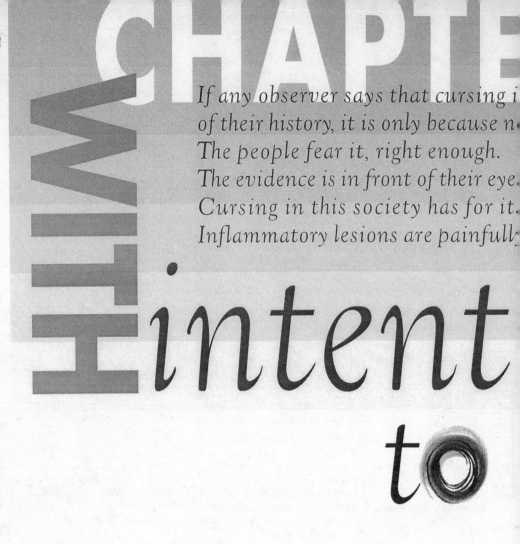

Skin sores and rashes abound. Deep wide ulcers—is it leprosy? you are bound to ask—cannot be ignored. Cystitis is commonplace for women, with miserabley scalding voiding. Burns and cuts are slow to heal, always hot and swollen. Sores and sorcery are synonymous.

In the hygiene-conscious West, inflammation is losing its place as the first and foremost chapter in the pathology book. Doubtless it is still the opening lesson in the classes provided in pathology labs in most medical schools. The medical student soon learns the hallmarks of inflammation as Galen[1] enunciated them: *calor, rubor, tumor, dolor*—heat, redness, swelling and pain, to which a fifth has been added—loss of function. But heat is the first. The part affected has been fired, as if with flame: it is inflamed. Where do those flames come from? Since the

ot rife among the Yolngu at this period
ody wants to talk about it.

nain aim the intent to inflame.
bvious and obviously painful.

INFLAME

advent of the microscope, microbes of one sort or another are incriminated. Germs have invaded and inflammation is the body's attempt to dispel the invasion. But in much of the world today this flaming heat is thought to be instilled by the evil of enemies, commonly called cursing, or sorcery. That is how most of the people at the Mission understand infection or inflammation. In the early days this was an understanding that led to a whole Gehenna of misunderstanding. People suspected other people of *raggalk* (witchcraft), *borrpoi* (poison), of malign and filthy tricks on one another, practised by cunning.

Attending to people nursing their

inflammatory lesions I came up against an infinitude of accusations of this kind, many guarded but others frank, detailed, angry and threatening. You had to enquire, because Yolngu are well aware that Balanda do not believe it; whites are obsessed with germs and fail to see what is going on! So I enquired, and I received some heated responses. The verb 'to inflame' is used in two ways in English, the literal way we have been discussing, and the literary way meaning 'to excite passions and emotions', liable to degenerate into violence. For Yolngu, the two meanings are as one, and they have the additional nuance that inflamed intent can be transmitted silently, secretly, dangerous and unseen, through the air around us, the very air we have to breathe.

Before we come to our case of an outstandingly intelligent man voicing some extraordinary—and piteous—pleas of cursing, I will relate how one of the oldest Yolngu in Arnhem Land, Thundercloud, explained to me how his people see this subject of borrpoi—how they classify it; how they perpetrate it; how they endure it; and how it affects their lives.

Borrpoi means cursing, the ragbag of poisonous tricks that Yolngu play upon their enemies—or even, as Thundercloud puts it, upon their 'unfriends'—in order to bring on their pain and sickness. If I were optimistic, I might expect that this description will capture the feel of it: the suspicion that nags, the worry that nauseates and the dread that makes the hair stand up on the nape of the Yolngu neck. But a description will not do it: if there is one subject with which Westerners do not empathise, it is cursing. People deeply imbued with the scientific cause-and-effect understanding of pain and suffering find the idea that other people attribute it to deliberate malice, or to evil spirits, is untenable, incredible and medieval. I know this from experience of teaching students; it strikes most Westerners this way.

Still, we are talking about exotic disease. If we leave out borrpoi, we leave out something that brings these folk to suspect, to worry and to dread. So let us see it the way they see it, for they mean every word. The way they pronounce borrpoi, all r's, so resembles the Queensland Aboriginal, Melanesian and Indonesian word puri-puri that I surmise the terms might be related. The concepts are the same. Your enemies generally proceed by taking by

stealth an item of your private and personal property and they elaborately injure it. And by harming this effigy, they hurt you. Thundercloud explained:

Borrpoi is the mixture of deadly things, killer things, put together to poison somebody. *Borrpoi* goes right through Arnhem Land, just as much now as it ever did. This poisoning goes from person to person right through the land. It has happened to me many times.

The main methods are *gundirr borrpoi*: poisoning with hot stones; and *dhupun borrpoi*: poisoning in the hollow log. If you perform *gundirr borrpoi*, first you steal the trousers or the shirt or the blanket of your enemy; then you rub it with the sweat of your armpits, especially hard on the crotch of the trousers. You can put on some of your urine as well. Then you dig a hole in the ground like an oven, and you roast those clothes with stones cracking hot from the fire, with a layer of paperbark to keep the heat in and some sand on top of that. You might put in some water to make steam. You bury it level with the ground so people don't know it's there. This will bring on *borrpoi*: the arm or foot of your enemy will twist, the skin will swell up and tighten, the belly distend with wind, or the mind go stiff and blind. *Dhupun borrpoi* is the same, but using a hollow log instead of a stone oven in the ground.

Here's another common way. *Ngal borrpoi*, spit poison. If I took a *mielk* [woman] from you, you lose her, but you are waiting for your revenge. Sooner or later I am bound to spit on the ground and you, my unfriend, happen to see me do it. As soon as my back is turned you take my *ngal* (spit) and roast it in the rock oven. Something strong may have to go in with it to give me real pain; it might be a lightning stone or a fiery stone from a sacred place. As well as *ngal borrpoi*, we have *luka* [hand] *borrpoi*; *kong* [foot] *borrpoi*; *dharmbal borrpoi* [on the mark on the ground where you sat].

Today I believe this is happening everywhere in this Mission township. But today they steal the handkerchief, dirty from your eyes and nose, or the old sweaty band from your wristwatch, or your bandage or even your socks. When one of those properties goes missing you can start worrying about your health.

The Balanda have brought the Yolngu some new and stronger ways for *borrpoi*. The acid chemical from batteries; this idea comes from the Balanda. Why don't you see Mangrove about this *borrpoi*? He's working in charge of the garage, so he knows how much battery acid goes missing. They spread it in your boots or on the seat of your vehicle. It's Balanda deadliness with Yolngu deadliness, together.

It goes further than that down in the machine workshop. Have you seen a tree which has two branches which cross and rub, the one scratching the other? This is called *dharrkaliny*; we use this place to put in your victim's patch of urine from the ground; the damp earth goes into the *dharrkaliny*. That is *dharrkaliny borrpoi*. In the place of that tree, some *dirrimu* [men] now find that an engine is better; the piston or the belt or the shaft rubs harder and hotter. So Yolngu are using machines today. They put the stolen clothing in the machine and let it heat and grind. Or they use the hot water tank: they secretly put something in the tank and let it boil forever. This is *gurrmurr* [hot] *kapu* [water] *borrpoi*.

Why do you think the young men won't stay for work in the garage? They're always leaving it! Sickness is waiting for everybody here, and we believe that much of it comes from the garage. In the workshop, they work for a few weeks and then they leave. Why leave a good machine job and run away? Because people wonder if some silly mechanic in there is playing about on the job, with *borrpoi* and *nyirra*, poison and songs, with their sweat, socks, handkerchiefs in the engines? Or even if he is not doing it, the mechanic worries that he might be blamed for doing it.

You mentioned *puri-puri* that you saw in New Guinea. We have *buri puroi*. It's a little different: it's love tricks. It comes from the Malayan people, we think. When the Macassans came to Australia, the old people believed that they brought a quickness and a brightness into the lives of the Yolngu people. What they brought to us was a new cunning: this was *buri puroi*, or love

tricks. They could trick anybody with this. They could use it to bring in a girl, or find a girl. They had mockery tricks, to mock the parents so they wouldn't notice that the girl was being loved. And then the poor man to whom this girl was promised would have to send out *nyirra* and *borrpoi* to make her lover sick, to bring the girl back. Or he might do it through spitting in the drinking water—the cup or baler shell. These things spread love between men and women too widely today. Through these happenings a *dirrimu* can lose a mielk or gain a *mielk*, or a *mielk* can lose or find a *dirrimu*. These are no miracles: they are ordinary events in Arnhem Land, every day and every night.

I demurred. 'Thundercloud, my friend, surely you are exaggerating about the machines? The machines around here work pretty well, if you service them'. Then I remembered that the lights had gone out last night, while I was writing. The generator blew a fuse, I surmised. I had to use a candle until the electrician put it right. Now, I had a sudden vision of what might have been the popular thinking about the same event.

Then I remembered that the magnificent modern bakehouse, fitted with new electric ovens and mixers at enormous cost, paid for by a government grant, was closed because nobody wanted to work in it. People preferred to have bread of an inferior kind flown in by air, at enormous cost. It was easier than operating the bakehouse. Or was it safer? Those ovens could cook a man's underpants to perfection, obviously. The bakehouse could be tantamount to the fiery furnace of hell, in the estimation of the people.

And I remembered Billabong With Ducks, who is the town barber. He does a neat job, of the length and style the customer wants. The customers, at the time of my visits, were carefully saving all the clippings and taking them home in paper bags. At home there must be a very large bag of it, which they lock away carefully so that nobody can practise *borrpoi* on it. Not so long ago folk would weave hair into string to make a sacred object, like a decorated dillybag. But trustworthy people with the string-making skill are rare. How they dispose of their hair I do not know, and they are not telling.

To our story.

It was a stifling day in December, hot to the point of mental paralysis and utter inertia. No breath of air stirred the motionless leaves of the parched stringybark trees. It was the kind of day you pray for a cyclone—anything would be better than this. Only the crows had the energy to move. I asked my companion, a distinguished elder of a distinguished clan, with as much exasperation as I could raise, if anybody knew how to call up a wind.

'Easy!' said my companion. 'The *nyirra* [evil breeze] or *djarada* [love breeze] are winds which anybody can make simply by mixing sweat from the armpit with crushed grass and throwing it in the direction of your wish. This will bring a wind and perhaps some rain. I'm not talking about real rain in a big thunderstorm, because that's the job of the Thunderman, the Dhuwa Ancestor Djambuwal or Larrpan. And beyond that, there is the mighty cyclone wind itself, the spinning wind which knocks down houses and pulls up trees by the roots. That wind is Burrmalala, which is a Yirritja Ancestor.'

'No,' he continued, 'I'm talking about the light winds that people can raise. This does more than change the weather; it changes the person it's aimed at. Women raise the love wind, *djarada*, over long distances or across a long time. A love song carried on the breeze. Arnhem Land women do it all the time. It fans the men and arouses them. And there are plenty of doctors, *marngits*, who can send a *nyirra*, an evil song to make us sick, a curse carried on the breeze. It comes from the power of your sweat: your wish goes into the sweat of your armpit. It's not only us Yolngu who do that. It's in the Book of Exodus. God told Moses to put his hand on his armpit. His arm turned white and silver, collecting the power; he stretched his arm out over his people and he controlled them with his sweat. It is the sweat of the body that brings a wind capable of carrying a message from one mind to another. It's like a radiotelephone—that's very like a *nyirra*, carrying a voice on the winds through the sky. The *nyirra* is especially strong in the wet season because they get extra power from the greater sweat.'

After this discussion of *nyirra* and the machinery of cursing we parted. It was too impossibly hot to work. Everybody rested and waited for something to change; anything would be better than such overcharged stillness in such unendurable heat. But in the evening my companion returned to talk with me. Our discussion must have kindled his fears of attack and reprisal by enemy Yolngu—an obsession never far from his mind. We sat in the blessed shade of evening while he astounded me with the heat that inflamed his mind. I was as astonished as incredulous at what he had to say: he hissed his fears into my ear.

'The Ranger uranium mine in western Arnhem Land! That's where my pollution is coming from. Those clever *marngits* [wise men] are using the radioactivity from the Ranger mine. The Balanda know nothing about this. I'm not so stupid. They are sending it here to the Mission on the *nyirra* wind. Why should I feel so sick if I am not polluted?'

He was adamant, and immune to reasoning and explanation. He was inconsolable, too.

'Those clever and evil *marngit* in those Western tribes are using radioactivity against us. Can I come to your hospital in Sydney? Can you give me a bottle of radioactive medicine like you use in treating cancer, to arm me against these evil people?'

In response to this, all I could do was ask the standard medical questions which every doctor asks patients, and to wait and see what came.

'How is it affecting you?' I asked.

He paused for a long time, then replied in a wistful voice, infinitely weary, yet confiding still. He was not yet bereft of hope.

'For the past two years I've touched no woman. Why has this happened? Who took away my life of sex? Who scorched it? Who stopped me going to the woman, and the woman to me? I took to eating trepang. I boiled trepang and ate it for a month. It did not help. I have some love magic from Borroloola in a jar in my suitcase. I rub it in each night. It does not help either. That is why I suspect uranium. Some Yolngu, my enemies, have stolen uranium from the mine and taken it to their *marngit* to send its pollution against me. But is it just against me alone? I wonder about that. I go around and I spy on lovers, men and women. While they love, I think I can see a green glow around their hair and their faces. It is the colour of uranium.'

His speech trailed away. I judged it

was time to offer a few medical observations, a few facts. I would not have troubled myself if I thought he was fixed in his delusions. I judged him short of reliable information, so I offered him some in as quiet and convincing a tone as I knew, addressing his fears and misconceptions. I am not sure just what I said but it touched on the obvious points.

'The uranium in the ground at that mine is very weak. It would not harm anybody. Only a geiger counter would know it was there. Those rocks must be concentrated, like a medicine, to make it strong enough to have any effect. A thief who steals some from the mine is going to be disappointed. It will not harm a man in any way. It will certainly not burn his testicles as you seem to fear.'

'There are two kinds of seed in the testicle of a man,' I continued my explanation, not too sure that I was being helpful. 'One makes sperm to make the woman pregnant. The other is for potency, for the erection that makes sex possible. Strong radiation might affect the sperm. I doubt if it would affect the erection. Cancer doctors know this and they are careful with their dose. The dose they use is too weak to harm the man's potency even if it harms the sperm. And I'm speaking about radiation from the medical machine, not uranium ore from the mine. That would scorch nobody.'

'Remember this also,' I went on. 'The sex urge leaves some men in their fifties. It goes. They lose it. Nobody takes it. Other men keep it until they are 80. With others, it sleeps and wakens. A great deal depends on your partner for it to waken. Some partners would rather it slept; they try not to waken it. Children today are potent younger. It's the better diet. Girls reach puberty younger. Their menstruation comes earlier. But it may stop earlier in the older woman. All these things are in nature. You need not worry that somebody is busy trying to scorch your desire with uranium. Maybe you are older. Maybe you are worrying . . .'

He took it in and thought it over. I did not know what use he would find for my opinions. I knew he would probably reckon with them: he had done so before. All the same, he asked me to procure a geiger counter to carry in his pocket, from my colleague at the hospital, the Professor of Radiology. He wanted to check to be on the safe side.

It seemed reasonable. I said I'd attend to it. I thought I knew something of his hurt. There is a bride price in Arnhem Land, a legacy of the old marriage system. A man makes payments over years to the mother of his wife-to-be, and to her family. He coddles them in two ways. He warns and advises about their safety, and he provides them with food, the best he can get, to strengthen his future bride so that when the time comes she will not be lacking in passion to meet his own. I thought I knew something of his disappointment.

When I next saw him a year later, he said nothing about uranium and radioactivity. I asked him about the geiger counter I sent him. He had lost it. He was not interested in that. But he had not lost his grievances.

It was Christmas Eve. He skulked all day inside his house on the edge of the township. He felt feverish and ill. He was hiding, making sure that nobody saw him or spoke to him. In the evening he called at my place. He was in a towering black mood but con-

sented to sit down. He was morose and taciturn. We had just started supper: my Kamileroi assistant from Sydney, Billy Reid, had prepared some buffalo steak with potato and cauliflower so we asked him if he had eaten and would he like to share. He said he had not eaten, so we divided what was on our plates to make a share for him. He toyed with it then pushed it away, completely jaded and out of sorts. Billy Reid eyed it hungrily but did not care to take it back. He was not impressed with his tribal brother's behaviour.

When he finally spoke, it was to ask if there was anything special for his projected visit to Sydney at Easter, meaning any special honour or recognition of his merit. When I replied that a break from the township, a holiday, was the intention, he was clearly disappointed and said he would have to think about it. He might not accept the invitation. We should leave the decision until March. He had wanted to bring as his companion a Torres Strait Islander from Sabai who was somehow living there, completely outside the kinship circle, while I had indicated a preference for one of the health workers for whom I could perhaps arrange some training. I was the one paying the fares. I thought his lack of enthusiasm to make the trip might be calculated to influence me in favour of his Torres Strait friend as companion. I knew he would not travel without a companion. But he would not have a countryman.

Then the full spleen of his mood erupted. He raved. It was those *Galka* at it again, making him ill and weary with their rotten filthy dirty tricks. 'We all know they do it. They bring poison to my system with their dirty songs so that I'm tired all day and I can't rise in the morning. It's happened a hundred times this year until I'm impatient. I'm thinking of buying a revolver for those *Galka*.'

My ears had pricked up at the mention of his inability to rise in the morning: that could be the complaint of a man with a clinical depression. But the announcement of the revolver drove it off my screen for the moment.

'Which clan?' I asked.

'Gumatj is one,' he replied. 'They think they should be boss for all developments. But there are others, all doing the same, worse than pigs . . . what is the highest and best animal?'

'The whale, I suppose,' I answered, with apparent innocence, for many people place the whale at the top of the animal kingdom, if we humans modestly step aside for the moment. Yet I did not answer innocently, for this was an answer likely to placate a man who traced his descent from the whale. It produced an unexpected response.

'Exactly!' he cried. 'The special brightness and superiority of the whale calls out the envy of the clans whose animals are lower than the whale! They envy my brightness from the scent of the whale. They envy my honours. Oh, the clans are still at war.'

He went on to talk about his awards and recognitions. All this should entitle him to respect. On the contrary, it attracted envy. It attracted malice and mockery! Yet here he was, fishing for yet more recognitions in Sydney, calculated to enhance his security. To most people there would be something unappealing in all this. He sounded like a policeman bent on winning a further stripe and kowtowing to aldermen, or an alderman bent on public honours, kowtowing to politicians. There was something

recklessly ignoble about such openness. There are things that a noble soul keeps to himself. He went back to the subject of the revolver.

'Who is the latest President of America who got shot?' he asked.

'Ronald Reagan,' I supposed.

'It's the same with me,' he retorted. 'I am being shot by the jealous clans. I need a revolver for *Galka*.'

'Nothing of the sort!' I threw at him. 'A revolver could never hurt a *Galka*, only a poor man, and then you'd never get over it.'

I had seen these displays of petulance before; they were nothing new. I grasped what he was saying. There were times when it might be hard to refrain from admonishing him for his want of gratitude, thereby adding to the censure to which he already felt exposed. I had heard depression speaking before, and this was its unsavoury voice.

I waited to judge the depth of the mood, to decide whether it needed medication. Meanwhile I contented myself with good advice, perhaps platitudes, instructions to ignore his *Galkas*, above all not to waste a gun on those who did not warrant it.

Clan enmity is in their bones, he had said; it was their world view not long before. The clans governed themselves separately. Our clan enemies have clever men who make us weak, or make us inflamed. Their songs are always in the air, aiming at our heart, our head, our nerves, our very bowels. Remembering this perception it seemed to me that my friend, far from being a misanthrope suffering from 'malade imaginaire', was merely honest. He said what he believed. He believed that the mockery he felt for his own worth was swimming in the air, clutching at his prestige, his importance, his very face. He was too naive to dissemble his grievances and to hide his hurt pride as a Westerner might have done. I made him take my antidepressant medication. Before long he was rational.

I suspect that some readers will not be satisfied with a story of cursing, but will want some resumé of this interesting subject, which is still used to explain the exotic diseases which concern us. Here is my understanding of it.

Sorcery (Latin *sors*, 'lot; fate') refers to malicious threats to life and health by an enemy casting spells. The dread of witchcraft, black magic and necromancy has gripped suffering humanity throughout history. These ideas remain as the predominant interpretation of disease and death outside the modern West. How did the idea of black magic, so patently contrary to modern ideas of causation of illness, become impelling, even universal? Contrasting interpretations are given by the social scientists, including anthropologists, who view sorcery from social and cultural perspectives, and by the biological scientists, including physicians, who tend to view it from biological and psychological perspectives.

From a social science perspective, sorcery has a logical sequence. Men who lack scientific concepts of disease, such as a germ theory of epidemics, attribute sickness projectively to the plots of an enemy. The enemy's magic, menacing, hidden, plenipotent, causes the infliction of pain and pestilence. This enemy must now be punished and so deterred. The task of the *shaman* or medicine man is to divine who the enemy may be, so that reprisal or retaliation may be meted out. In creole and

pidgin languages, this is what is known as the pay-back.

From a social science point of view, sorcery, therefore, is not necessarily 'sick'. Indeed, it serves society by making people careful to fulfil their social duties and obligations lest they offend others who may be capable of working sorcery against them. Providing endless gifts and services to propitiate people in one's social circle may be irksome, but neglect would lay one open to reprisals, especially to the malicious anger of those who may command evil spells. One therefore complies socially, and one works to keep pace with one's obligations. Sorcery's function, therefore, is to provide a stateless society with a machinery for law and order—this might be the view of an avid cultural relativist.

The rituals practised by sorcerers are invariably of a frightening nature. Exuvial magic involves procuring a discarded piece of the body of the person to be injured, such as hair, faeces, urine, nail clippings, or dirty clothing. This is known as 'taking dirt'. These dirty items are then annealed as it were with evil spells, wishes, incantations and imprecations. They may be roasted in a stone oven, or impregnated with hot substances, with the aim of inspiring heat (inflammation) in the victim. Projective magic transmits a foreign body (a stone, blade or bone) into the victim. Magical surgery is supposed to remove organs while the victim is asleep or in a trance, so that he or she dies in a few days.

'Voodoo' death refers to unexplained death associated with extreme dread from sorcery beliefs. If dehydration is not the cause of death, it is conjectured to result from a cardiac conduction disorder leading to a paroxysm of ventricular flutter and heart failure. This may be the mechanism of sudden unexplained death associated with extreme emotion. In the Australian tribes, dehydration is the actual 'killer', or mode of dying, according to the observations of my colleague Dr H B Eastwell, formerly of the University of Queensland.

The clinician or health worker usually has a distinctive viewpoint on sorcery, because of a closer knowledge of the victims. In my view as a clinician, the victim of sorcery has a more active role than was realized by the social science explanations. My study on Mornington Island, which I described in *Medicine is the Law*[2], found that in most of the cases no sorcery had been positively enacted at all. I found that a third of the victims were physically ill with treatable disease, but they explained it as sorcery. Another third were mentally ill, but similarly attributed their plight to sorcery. The final third were manipulating social opinion by accusing an enemy, hoping to muster resentment against that enemy.

As well as having a closer concern for the outcome of the victim, health workers tend to have a viewpoint that concerns public health. Where sorcery beliefs are dominant, it is hard to get a population to accept scientific explanations of ill-health relating to the role of hygienic or nutritional factors. Belief in cursing is not, of course, restricted to Aboriginal society: it occurs in modern society, but this would take us beyond the scope of the present discussion.

1 Claudius Galen (circa 130–201) was friend and physician to Emperor Marcus Aurelius in Rome. He was a voluminous writer on medical matters. He was first to use the pulse in diagnosis. He was the standard authority on medicine until the Middle Ages.

2 Cawte, J (1974) *Medicine is the Law: Studies in Psychiatric Anthropology of Australian Tribal Societies* University of Hawaii Press Honolulu.

WITH INTENT TO INFLAME

VILLAGE

I was tempted to preface this chapt[er]
thing the clans did when they cong[regated]
germ pool of inconceivable variety a[nd]
germ pools. Previously they had be[en]
waterhole or to a campsite, the su[rrounds]
visit. Now they were sedentary f[or]
pathogenic organisms which lay c[oiled]
I saw it happen and can describe [it]

under

Since no Yolngu saw this miasma of pestilence, no Yolngu clearly recognized that they were in it, submerged by it. It was not at this time 'our germ pool'. Yet its effects on their comfort and vigour were devastating. Infections were passed constantly from person to person, by direct contact or through aerosolized droplets in the air, on clothing, blankets and utensils, from contaminated ground or surface water or by insects. All this *reri* (sickness) affected Yolngu thinking, too: pain and discomfort were blamed, not on the real culprits from the germ pool, but on *borrpoi*, *raggalk*, the sorcery generated by a neighbour's spite and his malice. If a Yolngu suffered an infection, he did not ask himself, 'what?' He asked, 'who?' The answer came: 'neighbours!' Individual peace of mind and social harmony were thus equally

y a query: Micro-organisms or Micro-rapport? The first
ated in 1942 at the Mission on Elcho Island was create a
irulence. Yolngu knew nothing of insanitation, even less of
rotected by their mobility: by the time they returned to a
ind and rain had sterilized it from the previous
he first time in history, building up an arsenal of
ant siege to the body of each and every one.
o you.

SIEGE

threatened with bodily health. This was the sorry situation that confronted me around 1970 when I took the decision to spend my annual vacations donating my services as a medical practitioner in Arnhem Land.

Luckily, antibiotics had arrived in the 1950s at the time when both the population and its germ pool were burgeoning wildly, or matters would have become even worse. Several missionary nurses worked slavishly in the sick bays attending the stricken. But if cleanliness is next to godliness, the plumber is next to the priest and ahead of the nurse or doctor.

Yolngu and Balanda—black and white—were in tacit compliance with each other in some crooked thinking on the nature of the problem. Yolngu, who did not subscribe to the germ theory of illness, were unconvinced of the necessity for sanitation. Balanda, who were certainly informed about germs, underestimated the virulence of the germ pool mainly because they themselves were relatively immune to it, living as they did in conditions of superior sanitation and eating better food.

Among the others who might have been responsible for action, doctors were mostly absent; nurses were mostly

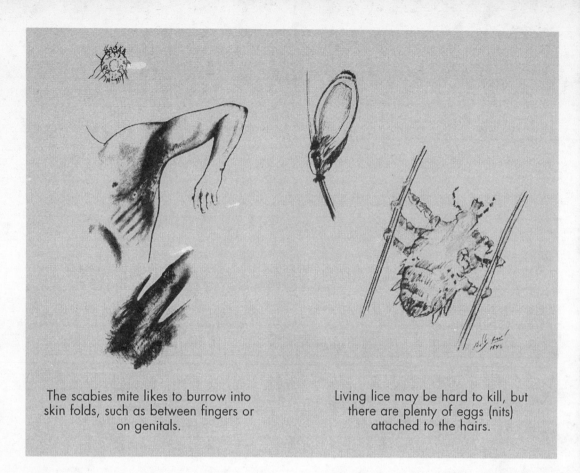

The scabies mite likes to burrow into skin folds, such as between fingers or on genitals.

Living lice may be hard to kill, but there are plenty of eggs (nits) attached to the hairs.

too harassed in the clinics; missionaries, teachers and anthropologists were mostly looking elsewhere. At the Mission, a dynasty of plumbers struggled to establish a sanitary domain amid a general lack of interest and money.

Yaws could not be described as a widespread infection, though certainly as an exotic disease. I saw two infants with yaws at a mosquito-ridden out-station in the vast paperbark lagoon called the Arafura Swamps in 1968. Pustules covered their entire bodies. Yaws is not a venereal disease, although the offending organism is a cousin to the spirochaete of syphilis. Happily, yaws in its early stages responds dramatically to penicillin. It has now disappeared from the germ pool, we hope.

Syphilis was itself rare until an epidemic occurred among the children at a nearby Mission at the end of 1975. I recall one twelve-year-old boy with horrid warts around the anus spreading into the cleft of his buttocks. He was only the twelfth child patient on Sister Jessie Smith's 'specific' list.

There must be a host of other infections I have forgotten, or missed, from this list of diseases less common in temperate zones. Of course, I did not treat at this Mission some of exotic infections of the kind that I saw in Papua New Guinea around the same period. Only sporadic malaria occurs. During my visit in 1975, two young men who had recently returned from Rabaul in New Britain slipped through the malarial net.

There were many other parasites and helminths, like filaria. Dogs, and to some extent cats, are host to some of these intestinal worms. They roam freely in the settlements, sharing places of eating and sleeping. They are hardly ever treated. Chemotherapy is improving for worms, but the treatment needs to be community-wide. Education and sanitation are more important than chemotherapy.

It was a struggle for the nurse to ensure that tetanus and diphtheria immunization programs were carried out and that nobody was overlooked. I always had the feeling that cholera was waiting in the wings for its cue. The relief from these infections was mostly due to the quarantine and immunization programs, especially those by

Here are some of the major infections I tried to treat at the Mission between 1970 and 1977.

Hookworm
Roundworm
Whipworm
Dwarf tapeworm
Leprosy
Tuberculosis
Poliomyelitis
Bacterial upper respiratory
    infection
Bacterial lower respiratory
    infection
Gastroenteritis and diarrhoea
Bacterial dysenteries
Typhoid fever
Trachoma and ophthalmia
Otitis media and externa
Influenza
Measles and other exanthemata
Boils; abscesses; furuncles;
    carbuncles
Scabies; ringworm; fleas; lice
Cellulitis
Infected wounds, burns and bites
Venereal disease, including
    gonorrhoea, syphilis and
    chlamydia
Yaws, chiefly on babies' mouths
    and mothers' breasts

the Commonwealth Department of Health, which were backed up by the hard work of the Northern Territory Health Department.

Let me recount but one battle in the war between the Yolngu and their germ pool. The 'battleground' was a woman called Blackfish. Just one case, but she can stand for the others, who thought their germs came from curses.

Sitting peacefully in church one hot Sunday morning I was touched lightly on the shoulder by the nurse, whose name was Kathy. Blackfish is in labour, or perhaps miscarrying, she said. I rose and found Blackfish miscarrying, haemorrhaging *per vaginam*. She was just alive; apathetic and unresponsive. She had not been near the nurse for any antenatal care; indeed she was not known to be pregnant. She always avoided the health centre.

Clinical testing then and there revealed the grossness of her debility. Let me take you on a tour through Blackfish's labyrinth of pathology. Her kidneys were damaged, leaking badly: her urine was loaded with albumen and some sugar. Her blood pressure was elevated at 190/140. Her lungs were full of strange noises and she had a chronic cough. She proved to be a heavy aspirin taker and tobacco smoker, using the Macassan pipe and the crab claw pipe. She was also quite deaf, with perforated eardrums. Her eyelids were scarred from old trachoma. I did not test her vision: she was not well enough for that. I judged that there was not much eyesight left.

But the most serious and startling hidden indicator of her sickness which came to light was her blood, or lack of it. A drop of it was watery, like raspberry lemonade. She scarcely had enough blood to keep herself alive, and not enough for her baby. I checked her blood with the clinic's new haemoglobinometer, a superior instrument to the one I possessed. The procedure involves matching a drop of the patient's blood, dyed green, against a green colour scale. Blackfish's value was four grams of haemoglobin per cent compared with a normal of ten to fourteen. Incredulously, I checked the gauge against a drop of blood from my own thumb—which came to a lusty sixteen.

Hookworm! Ankylostoma, the hook-mouth. I pictured a white swarm of blood-sucking threads, each with its mouth applied to a villus of her bowel, sucking her, draining her. I pictured minuscule eggs deposited in faeces in the mud by people who decided on that occasion not to add to a toilet pan that somebody failed to empty. I pictured Blackfish with muddy feet walking in the shade of a tree where people had gone to stool. I pictured the tiny larvae penetrating her skin and setting out on that strange voyage through her body to her bowel, where the adult ankylostoma suck.

We are told that when the eggs hatch from faeces in the muddy earth, the tiny larvae penetrate the feet and enter the capillary blood vessels. They ascend the major veins into the right side of the heart, which propels them into the lungs, giving the patient a 'wormy' cough. Maturing, they now climb up the major air passages of the lungs, over the epiglottis, down the gullet into the stomach, and thus come to their final destination in the duodenum. An astonishing Odyssey in the body! I pictured Blackfish, her head full of misconceptions about how and why she was sick, declining to come to the nurse for treatment.

Blackfish's hospital card contained brief entries which illustrated much of this multiple pathology:

1959	Otitis media, with perforations
1959	Hookworm treatment
1960	Trachoma treatment
1960	Diarrhoea—undetermined? gastrointestinal parasites
1961	Hookworm treatment
1962	Diarrhoea—undetermined ? parasites
1965	Urinary infection; heavy albuminuria
1966	Recurrent urinary infection
1967	Chronic albuminuria, elevated BP Sent to Darwin for medical investigation
1967	Typhoid fever
1969	Continued pyelonephritis
1970	Miscarriage at 20 weeks
1972	Continued nephritic state with elevated BP

Now it was 1973, and she was miscarrying again. While I was engaged in determining the nature and extent of her illness, she suddenly produced a 24-week-old foetus, dead and macerated, yielding up a miserable placenta without bleeding. She was hardly aware she was in labour. She was enfeebled, in and out of consciousness, getting ready for *Buralgor*, the spirit home in the east.

With all Sister Kathy's care and treatments, including worm powders and meat to eat, Blackfish began to revive and did not yield up her spirit after all on this occasion. A week later she could barely stand up, but she insisted on leaving the hospital. Hospitals are places where people die! I had about as much rapport with Blackfish as she did with me: nil. We lived in separate conceptual worlds, and did not understand one another.

The superintendent added some

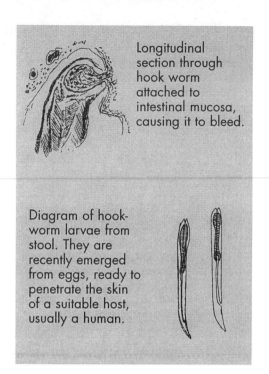

Longitudinal section through hook worm attached to intestinal mucosa, causing it to bleed.

Diagram of hookworm larvae from stool. They are recently emerged from eggs, ready to penetrate the skin of a suitable host, usually a human.

interesting information to that which I'd found on the card. It was Blackfish who was supposed to have brought to the Mission that disastrous outbreak of typhoid fever in 1969, having contracted the infection, he thought, in Bagot Settlement in Darwin. This epidemic ripped through the Mission populace with hundreds of cases. By order of the Health Department, the whole population was directed to take a course of chloromycetin tablets, specific for typhoid. There were plenty of residents who declined to participate, and at the superintendent's request a policeman was sent from Darwin to 'persuade' them. In the end they all took their medicine except—between us—the superintendent. Certainly 99 per cent of the 1000 population took the anti-typhoid treatment.

Meanwhile the Health Department closed down the sale of fish from the Mission freezing works for more than six months. The ban on the sale of fish was then lifted. After this serious economic challenge, the struggling fishing industry resumed, but it never recovered. I am sure that Blackfish never had the slightest knowledge of her part in the failure of this hopeful source of money, employment and morale for the struggling settlement.

I have outlined the case of Blackfish hoping to illuminate some hidden enemies to health. You could find worse cases—if you went to Ethiopia. In Blackfish's case I hardly know which affected her most—was it the hookworm, kidney or bowel infections, overuse of aspirin and tobacco or her own health behaviours and beliefs? There is a tendency for people to believe that because there is a little hospital, a pair of resident nurses and an aerial medical service, the health needs of an Aboriginal community are being met. This is the 'hospital fallacy'.

Let us ask Mr Ken Cantor, one of a line of hard-working plumbers at the Mission, to give us a running commentary on the problems of sanitation, while we walk with him around the township. A statistic to remember, as we talk, is that there are 110 houses for 1000 people—this includes the humpies at the beach camp in the count of houses. Mr Cantor ponders:

The worst part of town? Disposal from the school is the worst. There are 500 people using it: the toilets too few and the cleaning too little.

The next worst part is the bottom camp, where an outside clan now lives. These houses don't have water laid on. Only that little shed at the back does: it's the shower, the sink, the laundry for everybody. The lavatory is a pan. There is one of these ablution huts for each two houses. The water flows out of the drain at the back into that cesspool on the ground. It should flow along the trench, but do you know—it forms a sealing layer in this peculiar sand and it won't soak away. We've got surface water all over the town, and every time I send in a sample to the laboratory the report says it's loaded with E Coli. I was brave enough to send one in last week and the order came back from Gove: Boil all the drinking water! Most of the Yolngu won't do this: some don't understand the reason, and some say they can't drink boiling water. This surface water comes from the septic tanks and trenches, and it gets recontaminated by children and others who won't use the dirty pans in the toilets.

The only septic tanks which function properly here are in the Balandas' houses. The septic tanks where the Yolngu live don't work even if we can keep up the servicing. They're installed to serve five or six people, but ten or twelve live in the house: that's about fifty six-pint flushes a day. In addition, the water from the kitchen and bathroom all goes through the septic tank. That's an average of thirty gallons per person per day: it won't drain in this soil. It just won't drain.

So the main problem with the septic tanks is overuse. The pipe leading into the tank becomes crusted because the bacteria don't have time to work. The blockage works back into the houses. I'm constantly cleaning them out and pumping out tanks because the outlet won't drain into the trench.

If we can't treble the number of houses in the township we'll have to get away from the septic tank, and go back to the pan system. But the way we run the pan system here at present doesn't work either. There's a human problem and an administrative problem. There is a team of six men allowed $600 a week on a contract basis to collect and remove the pans and the garbage from the householders. There should be three working on the pans and three on the garbage. I've noticed that only four work on it, and they split the cheque. They have two vehicles, a tractor and a truck, which often sit around for weeks with flat tyres. They are flat now. Look at them—right there.

There should be a system of inspection to make sure these important jobs are being done. But no Yolngu likes to confront another over a question like this, and the missionary staff are fading into the background, and don't like to do it either. The official policy is *self-determination*. Some people call it *self-destruction*.

So what happened last week is that the Village Council, having taken over administration of the village, has now asked me, a white man, to supervise the hygiene. Maybe I can tell people to do it, they think!

Mr Cantor and I then inspected the tip for nightsoil and garbage, situated a hundred metres south of the bottom camp and a hundred metres north of the bore. Many pans were standing on the stage, untipped, gas fizzing, flies everywhere around us. I have cut Mr Cantor short; he had a great deal more to show and to say. He and his team of Yolngu hygiene men are planning to lick the problem, *this time*. Perhaps it will help if the Yolngu exchange theories of *borrpoi* cursing (sorcery) for theories of bacillus? That will take time. What the people believe is what is commonly omitted from the textbooks. I plan to highlight it here.

Exotic disease comprises a vast field and encompasses many disciplines; we used to think of it, perhaps misleadingly, as tropical medicine. Nutritional deficiencies and sanitation deficiencies underlie many of those exotic diseases. What keeps people submerged in this? Much of it is contingent upon what the people believe, and what they prefer.

Filth, from the Old English *fylth*, is hardly an exotic item. One can find accumulations of foul matter, garbage, debris, rubbish, wastes, wherever folk live together. Filth diseases are the fate of people who are condemned to live in it. Why are they so condemned? What entraps them? Why are they not free to clean it up or depart? We might have posed this question to poor Blackfish, who served us for our case of a person simultaneously besieged by a horde of micro-organisms. That is the intent of this book—to listen to what the patient says or disclaims, as well as to what the medical doctor propounds or proposes.

Blackfish said nothing. She was too sick and too shy. I treated Blackfish like any visiting doctor; I was not part of her world and we failed to reach each other. The most resourceful physician in the best-equipped dispensary would fail as I failed with Blackfish. The

physician must discover the patient as a person to make headway.

Blackfish and I achieved only micro-rapport. When she was well enough to escape from hospital, she would return to her way of life, believing that enemies were making her sick and curses were killing her.

When I slowly gained some grasp of the languages and personalities, and achieved some intimacy and rapport, I had more success with other invalids. My hope is that rapport will become as vital to doctors as micro-organisms, procedures and epidemiology. All are needed for the recovery of the people.

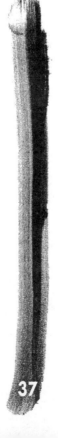

MARTYR of NIGHTSOIL

When a mining company undertakes
in some remote region it builds a comp
it makes ready is the water supply and
Safe sanitation is the miners' right; they
The company engineers are backed by
It was different with Aborigines and
they may have had neither.

There is a charming little freshwater lake south of Buckingham Bay in Arnhem Land. Harold Shepherdson, the aviator-missionary, spotted it on one of his flights and named it Lake Evella, after Eve, the wife of his missionary colleague Reverend Webb, and his own dear wife, Ella. Lake Evella is very small, but being a rare permanent freshwater supply it looked the place for a secluded settlement. And so it became; the church, houses, garage and store were established at its rim. A sanitation engineer would have kept this settlement back over the rise, where it would not drain into the lake and risk contamination of the precious water.

The main population was, and remains, at Galiwin'ku on Elcho Island. By the mid-1970s this Mission township had been established in its island fastness for some 30 years, growing steadily all the time, until it contained some 1000 residents. A road called

R FOUR

the extraction of a new find of ore

any township for the miners, in which the first thing

sewage disposal.

will not mine without it.

he capital and the know-how.

missionaries; when they established a settlement

Turtle Street ran through the central part of town, obliquely across the hillside, lined by 22 identical cottages constructed of iron and fibro, having two rooms each. More than 300 people lived in those iron cottages, serviced by septic tanks. But the tanks had never worked well. How could they? It was never intended that they should serve so many occupants. The name of the Yolngu hygiene assistant was Digging Stick, and to say he fretted about them would understate his concern; they were the bane of his existence. Digging Stick was stuck with an impossible job in maintaining those septics.

If we look for a moment at the physics of a septic tank—in itself a subject of inherent grace and dignity since the water closet marks one of the great advances in safeguarding the health of humanity—we can discover why these could never function. If 12 people using the same toilet each day pull five 6-pint flushes, this makes 360 pints of fluid to disseminate each day, excluding newspapers, cardboard, clothes and children's toys, all of which found their way in. This excludes kitchen and bathroom water, which ran to ground nearby. The septic action never had a chance against these odds.

Digging Stick fumed at the back yards of Turtle Street, forever flooded with septic effluent from overflowing tanks. The ground was befouled by stench, decaying matter, and was swarming with flies, like many another Aboriginal townships, or for that matter the shanty towns of Manila or Mexico City, where slum dwellers are too poor to pay barrio rates to have the human waste removed by the Sanitation Department. There was nothing unusual in this situation, nor in the communicable diseases. What was perhaps unusual about the dwellers in our township was that very few of them—a minority and without influence—subscribed to the germ theory of communicable diseases. For most, human detritus was somehow related to evil, to cursing, to black magic.

Yet every health worker knows that bacteria bubbling from the trenches of septic tanks can reach the air in the form of an aerosol, which can travel a mile on any breeze that blows. Viruses, too, make the same water-to-air transfer. But they are risking water-to-water transfers also: if a freshwater pipe is damaged it can aspirate septic affluent, and many a virulent virus can withstand the stoutest chlorination of drinking water.

This was Turtle Street of the mid-1970s. The denizens contributed to the health clinic more than their share of chest infections, ear infections, bowel infections and infected cuts and sores. Here the attendants worked hard with their dressings and their antibiotics. It must be emphasized that they also made heroic efforts to counter the pollution. But you do not get the same results that ratepayers expect and demand when they pay rates for the hygienic disposal of their wastes. Turtle Street people paid no rates, and endured their wastes.

So far as I could tell, some of the septic tanks were incomplete, in that there was no soakage pit, or none that worked. Sewage ran straight out of the tanks onto the ground where it turned into black slime, which had no capacity to soak back into the ground. It grew grass and weeds abundantly and prevented water from evaporating, so that mosquito larvae could flourish.

Digging Stick worked with the plumber, Ken Cantor, who had not long arrived on the scene but had already

concluded that septic tanks would not do for Turtle Street. Yet nobody was happy about the alternative, pit latrines. Ken then came up with a compromise, a water closet atop a pit latrine. He showed the Council drawings of how they would look. He argued that they should serve for up to ten years, but that provision should be made to divert the contents into a side pit. Pits exert a

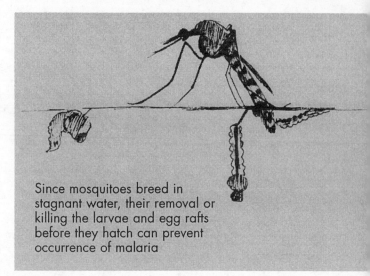

Since mosquitoes breed in stagnant water, their removal or killing the larvae and egg rafts before they hatch can prevent occurrence of malaria

septic action on their contents. The treated water should sweep away between the layers of the ground. There should be no contamination above ground. No flies, no mosquitoes.

All this was very heartening to Digging Stick. His situation as hygiene worker in this place was not an easy one. He was also pleased to learn that Ken Cantor planned to divert waste water from kitchens, bathrooms and laundries into a separate system. Pipes would take it into a manhole from which it would flow into a large mainline which would take it to a natural cesspool a kilometre away, to be purified by sunlight and aeration. The overflow would then go into the sea. No sewage would go into the sea. Digging Stick was happy about that.

I spoke to the District Medical Officer, Dr Joseph ('Joe') Caiquo, who came from Africa and knew a bit about waste disposal in villages. He championed the scheme. It could be paid for—a modest cost—from savings that the Council had made in its public grant from the previous year.

It looked as though the problem could be licked. And it was, but not without a heroic and tragic effort on the part of Digging Stick. Heroic, because in its way it was like the labours of Hercules in draining the Augean stables. Tragic, because Digging Stick was now harassed by insinuations and accusations from the people who saw reflections of cursing in his unusual willingness to mix with excrement and to excavate the earth. Each is an activity that incurs the dread of taboo. Digging Stick endured this doubtful reputation steadfastly until he achieved his sanitary goal; then he left the settlement and mysteriously ended his life, in circumstances that nobody really understands. I do not, yet I knew him well.

And that is the point of this story: it is the side of the sanitation saga that the engineering manuals and textbooks of tropical medicine omit. First let us survey the site, which I call Turtle Street, as the residents saw it, before we hear the details of these events and we extract the inescapable moral from it all.

'I find it hard to remember the street names in this town,' I complained to my brother, Stingray Spine.

'Baidi [it doesn't matter],' he answered. 'Nobody uses the street names, because everybody knows where everybody else lives. If you write me a letter, just the island is enough on the address.'

Notwithstanding this, there are signposts at every corner naming each street, and the names are distinctly long compared with their counterparts in a white town. I took out my sketch map of the Mission and indicated to him the block where I had been walking with Digging Stick the previous day, inspecting the marvellous new toilet system that had been installed when the occupants of the block retired from their houses for six months. The block was bounded by Riyalangura Road, Dutunggura Street and Marrpangdhangangala Street (which will show the *lundu* reader why I find it hard to remember street names at the Mission).

'I can help you with these street names,' said Stingray Spine. 'Riyalangura means by the spring, and refers to the spring coming out at the bottom of this road flowing onto the beach, which is why the Mission has always been an important place. Dutunggura means the *bunggul* ground—or ceremonial ground. All these street names were given by Djipandawuy, which name means Singapore. His name is Singapore because his father once visited there with the Macassans, and was impressed with that place. This long road here, around the cliff-top past the hospital, is Ganapay Parade, which just means cliff.'

'Marrpangdhangangala Street?' I asked.

'That is spelt wrong,' noticed my brother suddenly. 'It should be spelt Marrpanngurramangurra, and it means: Look! That turtle is holding something in its mouth!'

He picked up my pen and painstakingly printed the word, and drew a picture of a turtle holding an object in its mouth, so that I should not forget it again.

'I'll call it Turtle Street,' I said.

Now let me recount the story of the removal of the residents of Turtle Street while the new sanitation system was installed. I will tell it in simple terms, largely in the words which poor Digging Stick used when he told it to me, before his untimely death.

This part of our town was always dirty. The people did not use the septic tanks properly: they were always blocking them with newspapers, cardboard, rags, socks, underpants. Plastic bags were the worst. They never rot, and they block the drain completely. I tried hard to instruct the people, but they did not believe me about this. Some said they could not afford toilet paper so they had to use anything that came to hand, such as the plastic bags in which they carried their groceries from the store.

Dirty water was everywhere, with plenty of flies and mosquitoes. People could not walk around the houses so they never cleared the yard or cut the grass. They dumped their rubbish into the long grass. The Council gave people notice to clear the grass around the house or get out. They would cut a little grass, but the children would still throw rubbish into it. I talked to the people, and I tried to improve the ground by pouring on disinfectant with a pump, but it was no good. I was very sad every day. I talked to them but they just played cards afterwards, and they talked about me behind my back for a damn nuisance.

People were getting diarrhoea and sickness: because they would not use the toilets they would go to stool anywhere on the ground. Finally there were two with typhoid fever. So we went to the Council: myself, Frank Earl the head nurse, Ken Cantor the plumber, and Adrian Ralston the Health Inspector from

Gove. I think he comes from Ceylon. The whole Council inspected it. Adrian Ralston said that if it was a whitetown, he would close it down.

Everybody got angry. They laid it on the line. Suddenly the Council held a meeting with all the people. They said, 'We want everybody to move out of these houses! We will give every family two blue tarpaulins. If you want to camp on the football oval, we will put up some toilets and showers. If you go out to the bush, we will take your gear for you and cut the poles'. One third of the people went to the bush or the beach, and the others camped on the oval.

For the people camping on the oval we put up four toilets and two shower blocks. I saw to it that the pans were emptied twice a week. I collected the rubbish and burned it at the tip, so no food was left, and no flies were coming back to the town.

Digging Stick ruminated about human nature, or at least Yolngu human nature.

It's a funny thing, but in a bush camp the people keep it well swept and go to stool a long way off. Why not in town?

Then the whole town was given leave to stop work for four days. The Council had bought 200 jungle knives at 50 cents each from a Chinese dealer in Darwin. Everybody cut grass while the boys picked up tins, timber, logs, rubbish, old clothes and rusty pipes. Turtle Street was looking cleaner from all this hard work.

The contractor with the bulldozer came in and dug a large hole behind each house. Old toilets, septic tanks and pipes were pushed into these holes, and covered with 4 feet of dirt. When all this was flat, they poured concrete behind each house for the foundation of the new toilets. They left an opening 4-feet square in the concrete, and then we got in and dug a pit 9-feet deep. We cut the handles short off the shovels. It was hard work with those short shovels in those pits! At first the working men did not want to dig so deep, because they were afraid that sickness would come up out of the ground. That's where they thought their sickness was coming from. I was getting some nasty talk, let me tell you.

There were about fifteen men employed on this job, working overtime and weekends, because we had to get it finished before the wet came in December, and no more work could be done. We put up the new toilet houses, made of bricks on top of the concrete base, and then we connected the water to each toilet from the 4-inch water main. We connected every house and every toilet. That completed the toilets, but Turtle Street was not yet ready for the people to return.

For now we had to take away the waste water from the kitchen, shower and laundry. This did not go into the toilet, but into a big 9-inch pipe for waste water on the low side of the block. Pipes from every house ran into this main waste water line which passed along the lower road. These pipes do not run into the big pipeline itself, but into sumps which we can use for clearing and inspection.

This big waste water line runs along the road and then out into a pool near the cliff top. Then it overflows through a fast creek, which we made through the gravel down into the sea. There are no flies or mosquitoes in this pond because the water is running. But we have to burn off the grass all the time to stop the mosquitoes breeding in still water. That completed the waste water line, quite separate from the toilets.

While we were doing this sewerage work, the builders under Crocodile the carpenter were lining all the houses with fibro. They put in new ceilings, and cleaned and painted everything bright. They put in brand new electric wiring, new lights, and power points which they did not have before. The whole job took from March to October to finish, and then at last all the people could move back home.

This was Digging Stick's tale as he told it to me in private. Now let us tune in to some of the hints that came to the ears of this 'busybody'. Digging Stick was acting—as I heard it amusingly described—like the stool pigeon of the whites. Much of it did not reach his ears directly, he said, but was reported

to him by his wife. She took pains to tell him of the warnings that she overheard from others, and about the bad dreams that she herself was having. She was famous for her warning dreams.

In one of her dreams, the waste water that now flowed into the sea had enticed the deadly sea wasps into the Mission bay. Normally the bay has bright clear water over its white sand, and it is ruffled by the wind, so it is fairly safe from sea wasps in summer. Sea wasps like calm and murky water in which they can hide and find their food. Digging Stick's wife dreamed that the bay was now filled with calm and murky water and that the sea wasps were swarming in, stinging the little children who played in the water. Digging Stick protested that there wasn't any sewage in that water, and that it was carried away by the currents and the tides. It would not bring the sea wasps. But a deep dread gripped his heart. He tried to convince his wife that no sewage would reach the sea, that it was only laundry water with detergent in it, and no sea wasp would like that. She hardly wanted to believe it, and with her were the other mothers who feared the sea wasp for their children.

The big objection raised by the older men to the Turtle Street project was that their earth was sacred and that you should never dig it deeper than the length of a digging stick, as in digging for yams. Who knows what lies deeper inside the earth? For that is the place where the spirits of the dead, the *morkoi*, lie waiting for their release. The underground world must be left undisturbed. The mining companies were digging deeply in the earth: look at all the harm that came from that! Now Digging Stick was digging all these pits into the nether world—he was no better than the mining companies! They had no precise word to describe Hades, but Digging Stick seemed to be opening that kind of door. Sickness would come upon them all. It would be catastrophic! They did not confront Digging Stick with these fears and threats which reached him through rumour.

Digging Stick's wife claims that she dreams truly or honestly. If she dreams that a person is dying it truly happens. If she dreams of a poisonous snake or a spear, a death may occur. In the dream she takes great care to note the direction the snake or spear is pointing. They pointed to him, her husband, Digging Stick.

Now she said that she dreamed of a mangrove tree dying. The mangrove is the sacred tree of his clan. She would then get up sadly in the morning, knowing that somebody in the family was dying. She would dream of the tide going out: this also meant death. Or she dreamed of a rotting kingfish (a clan fish); this meant a death would occur. If she dreamed that the worms in the mangrove tree had died and gone rotten, this meant that a kinsman would die.

I tried to relieve Digging Stick's mind of all these omens of death. He said he did not take much notice of women's talk. He was at pains to explain how he could tell the difference between a true prophetic dream and a false one. If people go to sleep and dream of a subject which they have not thought about, or worried about on the previous day, the dream will be a true prophecy. But if they have been thinking or worrying about that subject during the previous day, it would be nothing unusual to dream about it. In this case he would take no

notice of the dream: it had no prophetic truth. People were worrying about toilets; to dream about it was not surprising and did not mean much.

Like his wife, he also dreamed of a spear or a poisonous snake as a sign that somebody was going to die. He also believed that if a cloud in the sky (not in a dream) takes the shape of a spear, it suggests that somebody will die. However, what he was doing was needed and was right; the people would see it one day and thank him.

In the meantime he had lost his friends, his social place. He still held his important post as the Hygiene Assistant but in other ways he was under a cloud, and called upon less to take his place in the ceremonial life. Less a man. People were waiting for things to settle down before bringing him back. He was too hot to handle.

For Digging Stick it seemed that death had two voices, speaking to him from opposite sides, in opposite languages, with opposite arguments. On one side he heard it: dig the earth at your peril for it is the home of the dangerous spirits. Leave shit alone, for that is the theft of the *raggalk*, the sorcerer who makes us die. On the other side he heard it: dig the earth into deep pits, for that is where waste belongs. Bury deep the shit, for that will save our people from sickness and harm.

Now we come to the resolution of the story, which I for one do not find mysterious in any way, nor even too surprising. We have very little reliable information on how he met his death, but we can conjecture the events. When the people were restored to their street and to their houses, fresh and hygienic, they forgot about their dreams and presentiments, and let go their irritable gossip to talk of something else. Their homecoming was in good time for the arrival of the wet: everybody was dry, comfortable and clean. It was as if they had never lived in a cesspool. They took it all for granted, as if it were part of the eternal arrangements of how human beings always lived in this world, ordered by nature rather than by human hand.

Digging Stick did not go back home with them. He left his wife, his family and his township. Nobody knew where he went or why. There came a rumour that he was living in Darwin with another *mielk*. I do not know the truth of that. There was also a rumour that he was drinking. I do not know: it is not unlikely. All I know is the police report stated that his body was discovered, drowned, in a tidal estuary called Race Course Creek near that city one morning, together with the body of another man. There were no suspicious circumstances.

I do not know if the township enacted the Morning Star pageant and the rites of the dead for the passage of that man's soul. He was a hero to me, a man who went against the tide of misinformation, indifference and prejudice. Paradoxically, I have some movie footage (which I would not show in public) of this man Digging Stick demonstrating in a jocular way to the

camera the essences of cursing. He is enacting the part of a *morkoi*, the forest sprite that is the harbinger of death. I sometimes play this movie privately, to bring him back, to remember what he did to help his people cross the hygiene bridge to communal living.

The Darwin coroner may have considered his demise in Race Course Creek as accidental death. It had happened before; drunken individuals asleep in the creek bed have been drowned by the swift incoming tide of that estuary.

I remember Digging Stick as the victim of those persistent prophecies and curses projected at him by his people during his work among them as Hygiene Assistant. Dangerous work. If one turns to the classical monograph *Le Suicide*, written by Emile Durkheim in 1897, one might refer to this death as 'altruistic suicide'—self-killing for a cause or a belief, like *hari-kiri*, reserved for men and women of samurai rank in Japan in a state of disgrace.

Farewell, Digging Stick. You are one of my private heroes, for whom I commonly hold more respect than for the celebrated ones. A martyr of nightsoil.

1 On my last visit, I found that plastic bags were banned on the island. Paper bags abounded. The people were not using traditional woven baskets of the kind I purchased years before, which would have solved this disposal problem.

LETHAL flu

The end of life is something less to be feared than to be accepted with equanimity or even anticipation. There are countless variations, but that is the general scenario.

Yolngu spend much time and energy on rites de passage, perhaps as much as any culture ever described. The deceased clansman is sped on his way with fanfare and éclat, in style and triumph. In Arnhem Land the souls wing to one of two offshore islands, the one lying to the east in the path of the tradewinds if you are quitting the Dhuwa moiety, or the one in the north in the path of the monsoon if you quit the Yirritja moiety. These islands are holding places of resting and waiting, something like the Catholic purgatory. Penultimately, the soul will take up its habitation in some natural object in its own country, so that the living are always surrounded by the dead. Ultimately, perhaps after many generations, it will haunt a man and a woman with *djarada*, the love magic, aspiring to gain rebirth as a living child, continuing the endless cycle of life.

The unresolved puzzle of life and death has preoccupied theologians, philosophers and physicians as well as you and me. The Yolngu explanation of it all fits their notions of power and the cosmos; their funeral rites serve to

ortitude with which the condemned Socrates drank his
e would have admired it even more if Socrates had
at awaited him. Throughout human history, most peoples
dy into an afterlife. The afterlife rewards people for efforts
id iniquities they have suffered.

highlight the solution and to reinforce it, concluding, as did John Donne, 'Death, thou shalt die!' Such views of death and the afterlife are of course congenial for those who are very sick, and for those who practise medicine, however much they are essentially metaphysical and liturgical.

In his bold essay *Beyond the Pleasure Principle* (1920), Sigmund Freud[1] examined the inevitable tensions between the self-preserving and sexual instincts, and the counter forces which lead to the cessation of all activity and to oblivion. Freud wrote:

This tallies well with the hypothesis that the life process of the individual leads for internal reasons to an abolition of chemical tensions, that is to say, to death, whereas union with the living substance of a different individual increases those tensions, introducing what may be described as fresh 'vital differences' which must then be lived off. The dominating tendency of mental life and perhaps of nervous life in general, is the effort to reduce, to keep constant or to move internal tension due to stimuli (the 'Nirvana principle', to borrow a term from Barbara Low)—a tendency which finds expression in the pleasure principle; and our recognition of that fact is one of our strongest reasons for believing in the existence of death instincts.

Freud's concept of a death instinct was coolly received by most psychoanalysts: it is hardly congenial for a therapist to believe that a death drive is prepotent. But it would not necessarily be discordant with the view of our Yolngu friends, in their rapture over death rites.

In order to highlight the place that death rites occupy in the health and adjustment of Yolngu, I can offer my recollections of a deeply evocative experience in which I participated in the 'Top End'. It occurred during a wave of deaths caused by an epidemic of virulent influenza in the closing days of 1973. In response, a tide of ceremonial activity swept across Arnhem Land.

In recent times, Aboriginal ceremonial (the 'corroboree') has been better appreciated by Europeans as a cultural expression of theatre, involving poetry, song, music, dance and painting. These art forms, seen by discerning eyes, merge into a spectacular total production, engaging well-trained and talented performers. Appreciation of ceremonial as an art form is commendable, but it neglects the question of its purpose and meaning to the performers. In indigenous eyes, ceremonial is a means to an end: it is conducted to safeguard the security and promote the wellbeing of the individual, and of the group of which he or she is a member. We may pose the question as to how successful it is in achieving this end, in the light of the ceremonial conducted to deal with this epidemic. I shall describe what I can almost call 'my' epidemic, because I suffered from it too, with fever and laryngitis such that I could not speak.

In Arnhem Land much of the ceremonial re-enacts the myths and stories of the ancestral creators with the object of releasing their power for the benefit of the performers, their descendants. By invoking the power of the ancestral beings, the rites are intended to preserve or to restore harmony, to resolve difficulties and adversities, to reduce tensions so that kin may live better together, to promote good health and relief from suffering, and to ensure plenty and fertility. Anything that may do that deserves the name 'euphoriant'. It surpasses alcohol.

My recollection of ritual activities is not so much that of an anthropologist as of a physician, flat to the boards with the sick, able to spare only a limited amount of time to observe what an anthropologist would have given all his time to. Two things stood out about the response of the community to that epidemic. The first was the extent and intensity of myth-ritual enactment. It staggered me. The second was the conflict generated by it, associated with the clash of values in a community which aspires to many aspects of modernity and of Christianity. Perhaps a good outcome should be mentioned: the positive relationship existing between leaders of the community and my medical team resulted in a movie film record being made of the funeral rituals. We titled it *Aboriginal Mourning*. This record will be of particular interest one day for anthropology. It illustrates, too, that white people are inevitably participant observers, in ritual as in influenza, whether they plan it or not.

It was later learned from the distant laboratory that the responsible organism was Influenza A virus of a virulent strain. Its spread, by droplet infection, from Darwin into the Aboriginal communities of Arnhem Land was undoubtedly due to the constant air traffic between settlements. (The amount of cash available is such that relatives frequently visit each other, and football teams regularly play matches 'away' on Saturdays.) The infection struck Maningrida, Milingimbi and Galiwin'ku townships simultaneously. Yirrkala, a less isolated community, was less severely affected. At Galiwin'ku, more than 50 new patients attended the clinic each day with high temperatures and complaints of aches and pains in the muscles. The respiratory tract was invariably involved, with running noses, coughs, sore throats, husky voices and, in those worst affected, pneumonia. There were three missionary nurses on the roster but they were reduced to two when a heavy flu hit the third nurse. These two women, assisted by a couple of Aboriginal health workers, toiled day and night coping with the epidemic demand. In my visiting research team I had a colleague who was also a physician, as well as my son Tom who was at that time a senior medical student, and we all helped with the seriously ill.

All age groups were affected by the flu. In the younger and healthier people the infection ran a shorter course, averaging three days, and then rapidly subsided, though many patients continued to cough and to complain of feeling weak and dispirited for some time. Older people and those already unwell from other causes were more seriously jeopardised. Antibiotics, intravenous infusions and oxygen inhalations were given where necessary. Aspirin and cough mixture were demanded by, and given to, almost everybody in the population of about a thousand. It must be borne in mind that this was a very young community with a small proportion of older people, the birth rate having exceeded 5 per cent per annum for the preceding ten years.

Four of the middle-aged or elderly members of the Mission population died, unable to rally from the virus because of pre-existing illness. One had lung carcinoma, another hookworm anaemia with furuncles on the legs, another melancholia with wasting, and the fourth senile infirmity.

For the purpose of the death ceremonies the community polarized itself into *bunggawa* and *djamamirri*— leaders and workers. This political structure is normally not evident in the village. During the epidemic the clan leaders quite openly assumed the authority to direct procedures. The followers seemed to accept this in a fairly complete and disciplined manner. (Important exceptions will be specified shortly.) This was in contrast to normal times in the village, when clan leaders are less visible than the elected members of the Town Council, only a few of whom are clan leaders.

The funeral rites were prolonged to an extent previously unknown in the village. At this time of year, just before the onset of the monsoonal wet season and at the commencement of the school vacation, the community would normally get busy with initiation ceremonies for the new group of boys. The age for initiation has been progressively lowered over recent years from the traditional puberty epoch to little boys of eight or nine. Now the initiation ceremonies were

postponed altogether in the face of more pressing needs for the control of sickness and death. Throughout the epidemic, the *bunggawa* appeared to work together in an integrated manner, originating and directing the ceremonies they deemed necessary.

The Dhuwa and Yirritja moieties were involved equally, two deaths having occurred in each, so that funeral ritual involvement might have also been expected to be equally divided. However, the two deaths in the Yirritja moiety were both in the Warramirri clan, so that Stingray Spine, as the leader, was heavily engaged. Now we saw little of him although, as my old friend and 'brother', he gave me what time he could, very creditably in view of the fact that he too was suffering from influenza.

Traditional funeral ceremonies among the Yolngu of northeast Arnhem Land have been described by W Lloyd Warner in his well-known book, *A Black Civilisation* (1937).[2] Since Warner's descriptions were written, modifications have resulted from the pressures of change, including the large and more static township populace, more demands of modern life and the influence of the school and the Christian Mission. Today, rites are performed chiefly by the members of the bereaved clans who are assisted by clans of the same moiety, with involvement in both early and late stages of the opposite moiety representing the mother of the deceased person. However, the sheer weight of numbers in the populace as it exists today makes a difference to the arrangements.

The dirges and wakes were similar in each death, though the crowd of mourners and duration of ceremonies appeared to vary with the importance of the deceased person. The proceedings were referred to as the *bunggul*, a general term for ceremonies. In all instances an awning was erected on a clearing of swept ground adjacent to the bereaved house, using for the roof large sheets of sky-blue polyethylene from the store—a cheap and durable material which has largely replaced tarpaulin in the tropics. After being left for a day inside the house, the dead body was placed in a conventional Western wooden coffin, made in the local furniture factory, and set upon a platform under the awning. At this time women took up their position surrounding it. Adjacent to the house, in the background, earth designs were made. These were excavations about a foot deep, covering an area as large as the house, of various shapes representing symbolically the clan waterhole in which the Spirit Snake and spirits of the dead reside.

The songmen chose appropriate parts from the epic song cycle of the Creator Ancestor of the moiety: stories of Djankawul in the case of Dhuwa, of Laintjung in the case of Yirritja. The dancers followed the song with well-practised mimes—of the crow, the seagull or the stingray—as created by the Hero Ancestor during his epoch on earth, 'in the beginning'. Most of the songs were brief, lasting little more than a minute, terminating with a rattle of the *bilmal* (clapsticks), followed by a brief rest for the dancers and sometimes a conference by the songman. As one song succeeded another, the ritual worked its way through the song cycle telling of the sacred places to be visited by the spirit of the deceased on its journey through its country to the assembly place of spirits and then to its sacred waterhole.

Most of the dancers had roughly painted—smeared would describe it better—their heads and hair, face, trunk and limbs with white clay taken from the cliff overlooking the beach, collected into tin cans. The white paint, it was suggested, stood for water described in the myth, particularly the clan waterhole to which the soul was being sent on its way by the singing. On one side, a few women swayed with small movements of their feet to the rhythm of the dance. When songs required their presence in the dance they came out in a body onto the dancing arena, some with small children on their shoulders, dancing though not mingling with the men.

As the *bunggul* proceeded, relatives who had been summoned by telegrams arrived by light aircraft each day from neighbouring communities, frequently a hundred kilometres away. The expectation that further relatives might arrive seemed to provide the reason for prolonging the funeral rites in order to give them a chance to take part. For example, on the fifth day of the first Warramirri funeral the truck was brought by the missionary in the late afternoon to take the body to the cemetery. The people attending the body were reluctant to let it go because, they said, another relative was expected on the plane the following day and they did not want to disappoint him. A long discussion ensued before it was decided that the body could be taken. The missionary, Mr Shepherdson, who was driving the truck, as a matter of courtesy took no part in the discussion. He was told that there had been a good deal of 'democratic discussion' (in the words of the clan leaders) concerning the proper length of this funeral.

During this *bunggul* at the height of

the influenza, the threatened rains finally came. The temperature fell sharply as the westerly monsoon blew full pelt and water fell in torrents from the sky. It came as a dramatic relief from the scorching oven in which we baked. In no case did the wild winds and rain interrupt the proceedings, however: the ceremonial continued with only short breaks, day and night, regardless of the thunder and lightning overhead. During this period some of the participants, clearly unwell from influenza, became very tired. Some were in fact exhausted, dragging about in a dull confused state of mind in the open rain.

An anthropological scholar may have noticed some of the respects in which these funeral rituals differ from W L Warner's early descriptions. Some adaptations are inevitable in a community living in permanent housing, using a money economy and sending their children to school. The most obvious change was the large attendance. With hundreds of participants and onlookers, the crowd spilled out of the yard of the house and onto the roadway, obstructing traffic.

The treatment of the body is much changed. In former times it was wrapped in paperbark and placed on a tree exposure platform—or in the Wessel Islands, in a cave at the foot of a cliff. Crows, putrefaction and maggot activity soon decomposed it, until after a month or two the flesh could be scraped away. The bones, painted with red ochre, could be distributed to relatives, ultimately receiving a second burial in a decorated bone pole kept in a sacred place. Since the inception of the Mission in 1942, however, the dead have been left undisturbed in the ground. Reports from Maningrida, a township to the west, suggested that the practice of recovering bones had been revived in at least some of the recent burials. But at this Mission the funeral rituals proper seemed to conclude with the Western-style burial, though they were followed by other rituals designed to purify and protect the living.

Before the bodies were taken to the cemetery half a mile outside the village, valuable objects were lodged with them in the coffins. The best clothes of the deceased together with new cloth material were put in. Old clothes were burned. Traditional sacred painted emblems, *rangga*, were laid upon the body, with copies of *maraian* (sacred) tools. The decorated dillybag belonging to the deceased and used in ceremonials was included. The Yirritja, the moiety which tends to ceremonialize innovations more than does the Dhuwa, put in modern objects such as tobacco, electric flashlights and money.

Instead of painting *maraian* designs on the body, the painters used the lid of the coffin. The large flat area gave more scope, and a good deal of time and care was devoted to it. These *mintji* (funeral) designs were not shown to the bystanders outside the funeral canopy. However, to indicate their presence in Yirritja ceremonies I witnessed, they hoisted on poles ten flags, including the Australian flag (a blue ensign at the fore) and others made by the women and oversewn with clan designs. They certainly lent this *bunggul* a festive rather than a funeral atmosphere.

When the bodies were removed to the cemetery for burial, a brief Christian service was conducted at the graveside for the close relatives who had accompanied the coffin on the back of the truck. These services are now often conducted by Yolngu ministers rather than by the white missionaries. None of those who were buried on this occasion were counted as Christians, but as one missionary explained, Christian burial services are conducted as an indication of charity. In a Christian burial a year later, traditional singing was sharply reprimanded by an elder (one of the *bunggawa*), as being 'out of order'.

In two of the ceremonies, the *bunggul* arena was deserted the day after the burial. This may have been due not so much to choice as to necessity caused by the depleting stresses of the influenza, the monsoon and the distractions of the next funeral. The final of the four funerals was that of Long Knife, who had been an important Warramirri personage. Long Knife never had anything to do with the Balanda; in fact he fastidiously avoided them, although he lived at the Mission. By the time his relatives decided to call me to see him in the course of his illness, there was no hope. I had no stethoscope with me so I put my ear against his labouring chest, which was full of rales and respiring forty to the minute. He summoned his remaining resolution and strength to turn his face away from me to the wall of his hut. I was reluctant to give him penicillin because it might raise false hopes, but his son ordered that I should and angrily told me that I should have come sooner.

In Long Knife's case the rituals continued in the same place in a modified form. He had had ten wives, six of whom survived him. These women were now painted with red ochre and became the chief object of attention. Songs were sung to ensure their freedom from their late husband's ghost, thus protecting their future health. Further ceremonial was then carried

out to safeguard them from 'persecution' in matters of marriage and domestic life at the hands of the anticipated claimants.

The second day was devoted in a similar way to the many children of the deceased man. In the words of one participant, the object was to free the sons and daughters from their dead father's governorship.

On the third day after Long Knife's burial, the ritual enactment became highly dramatic for those involved and for bystanders alike. This was a Yirritja *bunggul*, permitting introduction of elements from other cultures. For many years a large dugout canoe had lain neglected and broken on a dune near the beach camp. Children played sailors in the hull and visitors admired it. It was the only one left at the Mission from the historic era of the dugout canoe. It was a large one, carved from a single giant tree, with a beautifully shaped prow. The socket for the mast pole was carved from the same piece of wood as the remainder: there were no joints in the craft. In its day it had travelled hundreds of miles on the open sea from Caledon Bay in the east to Goulburn Island in the west. Since Long Knife had been one of its main users it was decided to remove the canoe to the *bunggul* ground outside his house and there burn it. Some of the pieces of the canoe were to be saved as relics for Warramirri and Gumatj people.

I was very upset about the destruction of this historic and beautiful heritage which I had long revered. Turtle Spear, who was of the Dhuwa moiety, a leading artist and prominent custodian of tradition as well as a good friend to me, explained that if he possessed a motor car at the time of his death, it would be burned unless his own son decided otherwise. He hoped this would console me. I was not so easily consoled by that. The people did not seem to realize that they would never create their own culture again. They were burning it.

While preparations were being made to burn this magnificent dugout canoe, ceremonial purification of the near relatives was proceeding. The men excavated a symbolic well in which they placed the relatives one by one and washed them with water to the accompaniment of more singing. It was explained that the intention was to get rid of the 'stink' of the spirit of the dead man. After the washing, those who had been cleansed were painted with red ochre 'so that the children can look at their bodies and feel sorry'.

None of these funerals resulted in any folk evacuating the cabins in which the dead had resided. Evacuation of huts and houses is still practised in other parts of indigenous Australia, for example, the Central Desert. But at this Mission this precaution against the ghost lingering among the living is not thought to be necessary. Perhaps the people are confident of the thoroughness of their ghost-speeding. And evacuation of the house would create inconvenience in a crowded community where more than twelve people, mostly children and adolescents, have to occupy the same dwelling during the heavy rains. Yolngu residents are careful, however, not to attract the ghost by uttering the name of its former bodily habitation. That might call it back. If somebody happens to have the same name as the deceased, the name is usually changed and the deceased is referred to for a few years as X's father or Y's brother.

'Value polymorphism' is a term used by my colleague in Canada, Eric Wittkower,[3] to denote the existence in the same person of sharply conflicting cultural values. He found that in the Inuit it is not infrequently associated with psychological disturbance. Although some value polymorphism is evident in many aspects of Yolngu Mission life, at first sight the ritual activity seemed to me to be consonant with or even supportive to the personality, rather than dissonant or divisive. This of course is the implicit intention of the rites, indeed perhaps of all ritual activity.

This 'consonant' aspect of Yolngu myth-ritual activity has been emphasized by Dr Nancy D Munn[4] in her commentary on Yolngu rites, as described by W Lloyd Warner. Dr Munn discusses at length what she calls 'the reversing action of the rites': the songs recall mythical events and the dances simulate them, and together they exert a reversing action on calamity. Communal ritual unites and integrates the people emotionally, generating an atmosphere of health and well-being for the participants and the community at large. Dr Munn writes, 'The communal enactments, in which the living Murngin [Warner's term for people now called Yolngu] identify with the myth protagonists, generate bodily well-being and food aplenty for all participants, by reconstituting the myth events within a controlling structure of social regulation ... The ritual repeatedly operates upon the events of the past to transform bodily destruction into health and well-being.'

Dr Munn observes that the funeral ceremonies are remarkably important in the ritual system as a whole. She suggests that the ritual cleanses death, puts it in the general system of meaning and relates it to the life cycle. She points to a preoccupation with death and bodily decay in 'Murngin' culture and finds it significant that the masculine role includes all the major activities involving sorcery, warfare and hunting. Munn's thesis is that the 'Murngin' myths convey body destruction images saturated with negative feeling, which the rituals convert into feelings of well-being. Thus Yolngu ritual, by this view, is a treatment of generalized anxiety by such mechanisms as reversal, catharsis and social integration. But I was led to conclude that this view may have to be qualified in modern times (and perhaps in traditional times too) because of the presence of some disintegrative or anxiety-arousing aspects of ritual. Ritual activity can have dissonant aspects, I found.

In this populace today, the best opportunities for myth-ritual are deaths and circumcisions of the boys, with the former more prominent. Marriage, an occasion calling for ritual in Western society, is not considered worth it here. Because of the privacy necessary for secret religious ceremonies, they do not conduct the Dhuwa *narra* and the Yirritja *narra* (men's ceremonies) in the Mission, so that enactment of these has in fact become less common.

Seeing that funeral ceremonies are so elevated in prominence, we should ask what their performance does to help the leaders (*bunggawa*) and the followers (*djamamirri*) respectively. I sought the views of my friend Stingray Spine on this question. His reply was given on 26 December, a few days before his brother died and he became more busily involved as *bunggawa* for the rites. I noted his instructions:

The two people of the Yolngu, Dhuwa and Yirritja, each have stories of the persons in the beginning, named Djangkuwul for Dhuwa, and Laintjung for Yirritja. These two persons were at the beginning of history, and Yolngu duplicate things from them down ages to ages. The Dhuwa duplicate things from Djangkuwul, Yirritja from Laintjung.

The purpose of having separate myths is to keep Dhuwa and Yirritja separate. Each is performed by different acts of dance, different songs, with different languages which developed as the population broke away from each other. This custom can stay firm for the future, and can represent the mala [clans] in Northern Territory and Australian culture. The bunggul furnishings, the proud design of the ritual performance of the myth, are made of red and white clay, of bark paintings, of the yirrdaki [pipe], bilmal [clapsticks] and the leaves of trees.

The Garma is the name for the public ceremonies that women and children can share; the Narra is the private one for men alone.

There are many occasions for the ceremony to be performed, and the law man mediates to decide if a ceremony is wanted. A funeral is one. A circumcision is another—the law man decides whether the young boy of eight or nine is big enough for initiation and good behaviour. Then he says he will put it on at the bunggul. A Kunapipi is another, so is a Marndiella—these are private ceremonies for special purposes.

All future ceremonies will probably be in the township. It is too expensive to go out to hold them elsewhere. And you can't hold the Narra ones in the town. And they will have to be changed because there is mockery on both sides, Yolngu and Balanda. Turtle Spear was teaching the myths in school, through painting, dance and song, paid as a teacher. He pulled out of this because he was too much in demand and never in one place for long enough.

Today there are two educations and two happinesses: if a man is not happy on the Yolngu side, he can go over to the Balanda.

In his comments of 'mockery on both sides' and 'the two happinesses' Stingray Spine is picturing a value dissonance inherent in the ritual. But from the *bunggawa*'s point of view, funeral rites provide an important opportunity for him to emerge from his relative obscurity and openly to exert his authority. The *bunggawa* men obviously appreciate the opportunity to display leadership and guidance, frustrated as they are from achieving leadership positions in a modernizing community, positions requiring more literacy.

The *djamamirri* (followers, workers or servants) seemed to be involved as well as wanting to be involved. Most of them painted each other with white clay. Spears emerged in profusion—not long before it had been made illegal for obvious reasons to hold them in the Mission—together with decorated clubs, headdresses and dillybags. Even the schoolboys now on their Christmas holidays were actively involved, copying their big brothers in the dances at the *bunggul*. There was a busy stream of traffic to and from the *bunggul* as some groups performed and others watched. They were all coughing and spitting from the flu, dragging about.

Many of the women, especially the relatives of the deceased, were also conspicuously involved in the *bunggul*. Early in the rites some women, taking a central position in the throng, gashed their heads with rocks to make the blood flow, seemingly relying on the male bystanders to restrain them if they should injure themselves too severely. One woman in fact did need her scalp stitched up—and I was obliged to do it. However, others inflicted symbolic wounds on themselves with a practised action calculated to 'hold the punch'. As the *bunggul* progressed, a few women showed their interest by dancing quietly and modestly on one side, and many of them came forward when the ceremony required them.

Some dangerous events occurred during the *bunggul*, mostly associated with the drinking of liquor. The Mission is officially 'dry' by order of the all-Yolngu Town Council. The effects of liquor are generally feared in the community. Several prominent citizens abide by an arrangement whereby they drink if they visit Nhulunbuy or Darwin, the nearest towns with hotels. They actively oppose liquor coming into the Mission. However, liquor is smuggled in at the airstrip under the nose of the Council's Yolngu policeman by influential citizens whom he does not have authority to challenge.

During the first funeral some argument came up about the rites, particularly their proper duration. In the very early hours—it was around 3.00 am—of the third morning, two relatives, who were said to have been drinking, snatched the body from the coffin and dumped it on the ground away from the house. Aghast at this desecration, the mourners threatened them with spears and the son of the deceased went into the house and brought out his rifle. It was hard to get a clear idea of the motives of the two men and harder to understand how they had been permitted to go as far as they did. Most of those whom I questioned purported to be satisfied with the explanation that the men had been drinking, and that drinking Yolngu do crazy provocative things, without responsibility.

Another dangerous incident occurred during the fourth funeral while I was watching. A young man, who was dancing with what struck me at the time as style and enjoyment, suddenly broke off and flew into a wild rage. It seemed to be in response to a remark addressed to him by the songman. He hurled his spear thrower over the house and his dillybag at the songman. Rushing to one side, he picked up a fishing spear and attacked another man remonstrating with him. A group immediately surrounded him and by some quick reflex somebody was able to grasp his spear from behind and snap the shaft in two. But the descending prongs delivered a blow which gashed the face of Wandjuk Marika, a senior and respected visitor from Yirrkala, who was one of those trying to interpose. The prongs scored the skin of Wandjuk's chest. Disarmed, the attacker screamed abuse for a short while then suddenly started to weep, standing by himself forlornly embracing a post of the house. Several senior men prowled angrily about with their spears fitted to their spear throwers, wanting to be placated by the others.

Wandjuk elected to come away to my house for medical attention. A cup of tea and a bandage were all that proved necessary, though Wandjuk's eye had escaped narrowly. He had been lucky. However, his absence had the effect, no doubt calculated, of delaying the proceedings. Wandjuk explained to me that the young man had been carried away by his own dancing and had started to dance 'individually', as occurred at Balanda 'rock and roll' dances; individuality is never permitted by Yolngu. Thus he was guilty of conceit and perhaps even blasphemy. When reprimanded he lost his temper. In former times he would not have been reproached, but promptly speared. Wandjuk said the man was let off lightly because he had been drinking and this made him mad, not responsible.

Perhaps the most obvious focus for Wittkower's value dissonance idea was the conflict between traditional observances and the ideas of the Mission, which are now shared by the younger councillors to a considerable extent. All through the funeral rituals, criticisms were being levelled that they were too prolonged. There was concern also about the number of spears that were being flourished around the village. Some people expressed irritation that the preoccupation with funerals had brought all normal work to a halt. Another concern was that most of us were really out of our wits with the flu and should be resting, out of the rain. We were all soaked to the skin.

It was indeed true that nobody was showing any interest in clearing up the rubbish and blocked drains, and the hygiene of the village was at the lowest ebb for a long time. I felt bound to advise the Council that it had good reason to be concerned about an outbreak of gastroenteritis coming on top of the influenza, but the Council seemed unable to do anything.

A heated discussion developed about the propriety of keeping bodies lying about so long before burial. My medical team itself was divided in opinion as to whether the preference of Western society for prompt burial is an ethnocentric attitude or based on sound public health reasons. It was recalled that in English villages within living memory, bodies were often left for 12 days before burial. I had just medically attended a Yolngu woman who had died. I found her to be severely anaemic, with a haemoglobin level of 8 grams percentage, compared with the normal 12 to 13 grams percentage. She had boils all over her legs. I doubt that any public health official would have condoned this body lying around in such heat. The boils had burst open to the flies.

In fact all the bodies quickly decomposed, and attempts were made to cover the stench by sprinkling them with deodorant powder. Stingray Spine was delighted to find a pressure pack of spray from the store, which advertised its contents in clear lettering: 'MUM 21-Body Freshener.' He was spraying this on the bodies, armpits and all. He asked why I was laughing. 'Wawa, Lundu,' I said. 'Brother and Friend, I laugh to save me from crying.' I did not actually say it; I croaked it inaudibly, because the laryngitis from the wretched flu had robbed me of voice.

It had to be remembered that the community was debilitated not only by the influenza epidemic but by chronic hookworm infestation, and by an indifferent diet of fast food. The fishing boats which normally supplied fish had all broken down or been destroyed by shipworm, and replacements were not expected. The community relied almost completely on the store for food, from which they mainly chose flour and sugar. A missionary expressed misgivings about this concentration on wakes, vigils, and funeral rites while nobody went crabbing, oystering or fishing.

On the other hand, the people were bringing out their herbal remedies in profusion. If I'd had the time or interest, I could have made quite a collection of plants thought to have medicinal properties. I was interested in psychosocial dwarfism (there was a scattering of little people there) and I could observe the severe nutritional breaks that can be experienced by luckless infants at times such as these.

Several of the younger councillors were talking of the need to make a law to restrict future funerals to three days. Stingray Spine, in a discussion before I left, asked me whether the coroner in Darwin, or the Old Testament, had a law about time before burial. I did not know. I said everybody had different ideas about the treatment of bodies. But then he recalled that a refrigerated mortuary had recently been installed in Nhulunbuy and could be used by Yirrkala residents. Perhaps one should be installed at the Mission? He would ask the government to provide the cash.

It was a moving experience to witness the conflicts of people without adequate experience of such matters being required to live together under township conditions. In time, perhaps clearer awareness of the work needed to achieve urban living would set limits to traditional ritual. That time seemed a good way off to one who saw this community reacting to the stress of a lethal influenza epidemic, extending its rituals with the fervour and euphoria of a nativistic movement. But then the Town Council had been in existence for only a short time—less than a year—and my experience had given me a great respect for the unusual adaptive capacity of this Yolngu bloc of Aborigines.

Tribal people who live in the remote reaches of Australia, sometimes sick, confused, aggrieved, still appeal for relief from every source of traditional power. An intensification of ritual activity arises to meet an unprecedented need. This resurgence of tradition will not endure, however, as the old ways die out and the new ones surge in.

1 Freud Sigmund (1920) *Beyond the Pleasure Principle* . The Hogarth Press Standard Edition 1955.
2 Warner W L (1937) *A Black Civilisation: A Social Study of an Australian Tribe* Harper & Bros New York.
3 Wittkower E (1969) Perspectives of Transcultural Psychiatry *International Journal of Psychiatry* 8 (5) pp 811–24.
4 See Marie Reay (ed) (1964) *Aborigines Now* Angus and Robertson Sydney.

CHAPTER NOMADS or wand

The Macquarie Dictionary provides

'1. One of a race or tribe without fixe

state of pasturage or food supply.

2. Any wanderer.'

The term 'nomadic' is conventional

They do however throw up some war

What on earth is up with them? The

As often as not, the reasons for their

I fear that two 'wanderer' diseases to emerge are generally unmention-able: schizophrenia and leprosy. These diseases are the doctor's business! Sometimes I have formed continuing ties with these 'odd ones', and they with me, so I speak about them with some understanding.

Here is a fascinating account of a young Yolngu jointly beset by leprosy and wanderlust. We shall call him Yawirongga, which is nothing like his true name. The story of his wanderlust came to fascinate as much as his leprosy, because it sheds a particular light *uble definition of nomad:*

ode, but moving about from place to place according to the

plied to Aboriginal tribes—which rarely have wanderers.

ers; they are commonly referred to me, as the doctor!

anderers are only loosely attached to the main group.

chment, or rootlessness, are medical.

erers

on the little universe of the Aboriginal reserve of Arnhem Land. This is an unspoiled part of Australia, with very few white people living in it and no roads passing through. No tourists! The coastline—as the reader may judge from the map—is extraordinarily intricate, with numerous bays, promontories, shallows uncovered by tides and offshore islands. For a traveller, or wanderer such as Yawirongga, Arnhem Land is full of enticing, remote corners.

I hope the reader will be as intrigued by Yawirongga's wandering as I have been.

Leprosy commonly represents two afflictions: the chronic disease and the equally chronic social stigma. The bacterial agent responsible for the infection, *Mycobacterium leprae*, invades the cooler parts of the body, notably the skin, the eyes, the more outlying reaches of the nerves of the limbs, and the testicles.

During my medical lifetime, effective chemotherapy at last confronted and halted this age-old disease. The most commonly used preparation is dapsone (diamino-diphenyl-sulphone, or DDS) which is a safe, stable and inexpensive drug. There are other drugs for dapsone-resistant patients, but in most cases dapsone works slowly but surely, and the disease is arrested. Nowadays, all patients in Australia receive multi-drug therapy, which kills the bacillus.

Once the disease is arrested, the surgeon can correct the disfigurements and deformities that have occurred through injury, because the hands, feet and eyes have been made insensitive to pain by the nerve damage. These injuries are common because victims of leprosy do not suffer the usual surface pain, and may fail to remove external parts out of harm's way, such as a fire that is too close. They are burned without knowing it.

The stigma of leprosy is traditionally rivalled only by the stigma of psychosis, that is, active schizophrenia or mania, which are also stigmatized as unholy and loathsome afflictions—the work of the Devil. Some people trace this leper's stigma to the Old Testament and to the Judaic laws and traditions about what was thought to be leprosy. In many cases this included other skin diseases, since diagnosis was anything but accurate. A multitude of sufferers of other obscure diseases were accused of ritual uncleanliness and cast out from society.

In more recent times the medical profession has done its best to reduce the stigma. It first abandoned the term 'leper' for 'leprosy patient'. Many centres then abandoned the term 'leprosy' for Hansen's disease, after Dr Hansen of Bergen who first saw the bacillus in 1873 when he examined scrapings from a Norwegian patient under his microscope. From this it will be readily inferred that leprosy is not always a tropical disease or an exotic disease. It seems that way today because over half of the patients live in Africa and India, but essential factors may concern hygiene and housing rather than climate or heat. More spacious sleeping quarters have played the biggest role in reducing the prevalence of leprosy. There is no other reasonable explanation for the virtual disappearance of leprosy in Europe after the Middle Ages, and from Scandinavia early this century, well before the arrival of chemotherapy. Where people still huddle in crowded quarters, leprosy remains endemic.

Nor is the stigma limited to countries that read the Bible; China also stigmatized people with conditions considered to be leprosy. The stigma in the West remains most abhorrent in the minds of those who derived their ideas about leprosy from the romantic tales of Jack London, Robert Louis Stevenson and Sir Arthur Conan Doyle. Not that their stories are inaccurate, merely outdated in the light of modern drugs and our insight that the disease seems to be transmitted when too many people are sleeping too closely together. I have had many leprosy patients with me in the field. They ate at my campfire and my table and it never occurred to me to think that I was at risk. But we never had to share wet weather sleeping quarters, crowded under a confining roof to keep out of the rain.

During the two decades that I visited the folk at the Mission, between 5 and 7 per cent of them would have been victims of leprosy in one form or another. This is the estimate of Dr John Hargrave. He wrote an instructive book about leprosy, with colour photographs.[1]

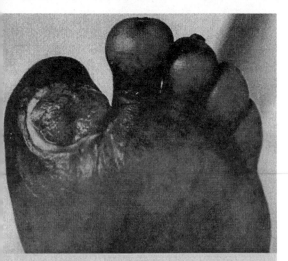

A leprous ulcer on the foot.

It mostly occurs in mixed forms and its rapid progress is now arrested by chemotherapeutic treatment.

I have read somewhere that although Aboriginal people suffer a lot of leprosy they do not stigmatize it. That is nonsense; whoever wrote it did not care to listen very closely. Some people, particularly those who are most attuned to sorcery, stigmatize it with thoughts of pay-back. Others, especially those patients who have been under the care of Dr Hargrave at the East Arm Hospital near Darwin, are less affronted. My inference is that Dr John Hargrave, as the leprology specialist for the Northern Territory, has himself done much to temper the stigma by his own close attention and commonsense. A physician destigmatize leprosy? The case that I will offer supports this claim. But there is one further matter we must understand. The people dread pay-back more than stigma and deformities.

Yolngu use the same word for leprosy, *borrpoi*, as they use for pay-back. They also use *borrpoi* for tinea, which is extensive and easily confused with leprosy by the inexpert. We shall come to that in a moment.

Yolngu did not derive leprosy from Balanda, the European invaders. It was first noted in the arrivals from Asia to Darwin at the end of the last century, and it soon spread out among the various tribes. Yolngu recognize several forms: they are all identified in terms of curses and pay-back, as I shall describe.

By their designation, *burundiya* is the form on the skin and the flesh. The flesh has gone rotten, swollen so the people cannot walk. It is caused by spearing the footmarks of your enemy. The story is rife that a bone from the skeleton of a dead person is the deadly spear to point at a healthy man or woman, to give them *borrpoi* pain or sickness. People often died of the *borrpoi reri*, or leprous sickness. The curse is divined by the *marngit* or medicine man: this man died because that man pointed a dead man's bone at him. This kind of death was common because if anyone offended, for example stole a woman, it had to be 'balanced'. The debt had to be paid back in full. This obligation was called 'pay-back'.

Duwal-duwal is the form that destroys the bones. If a Yolngu has done something wrong, such that his opponent wants to kill him or poison him by *duwal-duwal*, he draws his image on a certain tree and then rubs poison on this image. Some trees are 'savage'; they should not be touched or eaten; but if people are starving they are likely to take the wrong food and are poisoned. *Duwal-duwal* means the poisonous food, but it also means the disease of the bone caused by an image or effigy engraved on the poisonous tree.

Since some of my personal friends suffered from leprosy, I enquired among them and their peers what is generally believed about the cause of their illness. I was told that Marrayila's leprosy came from Doindji way, in the Wawilag area. Marrayila's father was Pangata, who killed an important Dhuwa man. That man's relatives at first planned to kill his family, but they had a change of heart, and simply drew a portrait of the son, Marrayila, on the rocks in a very powerful poisonous cave in that country. That portrait was his effigy, bringing harm.

Yawirongga got his *borrpoi*, or *burundiya*, in the same kind of way, I was told. His father, Djilirri, was said to have speared two people. One was Djambapuynu clan and the other was Barr-Barr clan. Instead of Djilirri, his own son Yawirongga got the pay-back.

So leprosy is a form of pay-back for doing something wrong? That was the general belief, now being questioned. I asked Dr John Hargrave to talk to this young man Yawirronga, to find out just what he thought about it. Dr Hargrave joined me at the Mission on numerous occasions. For many years we had Christmas dinner at the table of the founding missionary Harold Shepherdson and his wife Ella. John responded warmly to my suggestion that we needed the story of one of his patients, expressed in the patient's own words. I offered some guidelines. How does leprosy affect its victim's life? How does it affect his thoughts, his feelings, his coming, his going, his giving, his taking, his being? How does his attitude to it affect the trajectory of the disease and compliance with the treatment? Yawirongga's story, as told to Dr Hargrave, answers some of these questions. According to Dr Hargrave, Yawirongga is happy for us all to know his story; it is there for us to read with his compliments—if it will help us understand.

Yawirongga was born about 1943.

He was admitted to Channel Island Station near Darwin in February 1955 with lepromatous leprosy. He had sensory loss in his hands and feet, and in the left leg up as far as the knee. His smears became negative and he responded to treatment. But he had to continue with sulphones for a very long time, as the chances of relapse are greater in those who do not. Unfortunately it was not always possible to ensure that he took his tablets and wore his shoes. At least the conventional need for pay-back seems to have been dramatically reduced by his exchanges with Dr Hargrave. The cost of his cure was a personality change. He was institutionalised and dissocialised, as we shall learn.

Yawirongga's story, as told at the Mission on 29 December 1972

I was born in the camp at Marchinba, which is a place in the Wessel Islands. My father's name is Djilirri and when I was at Gurindin [Quarantine] I heard that my mother had passed away. When I was a young fellow I did not like school. All the time I was running away from school. My father had four wives as far as I know, and I am a son from the second wife. The same mother and father have these children: Marrayila, Walangitj, me and Yanamany, and one boy who dies. I had sores all over me and I didn't know it was leprosy. So I didn't know what leprosy was and he (my father) brought me to the Mission. He brought me back from Mata Mata and he wanted me to stay here at Elcho Island and get treatment but I didn't like it so I went with other people, back to Mata Mata where my father was. He brought me back a second time to the Mission and then the doctor came. The pilot was Jack Slade and the doctor was Dr Raiment. My father told me it was burundiya. That means 'sores that take a long time to get better.' [It has another meaning: a tree that is rotten and worm-eaten.]

When my father told me I had

burundiya, well, I just felt too sad and sorry for myself. I said to myself: 'Why did this burundiya have to pick on me?' I decided that if the doctors come and ask me then I will just go with them. Really I was frightened to go to that place called Gurindin [Quarantine] because I have never been anywhere. I was thinking I might die because I had this borrpoi burundiya [leprosy]. Darawa [plenty] fellows die before. I went on the aeroplane from here [the Mission] to Darwin and from Darwin on the boat. I stayed two weeks in 'boratory' hospital [Darwin Hospital]. At first I was frightened because I didn't know nobody there. They took me down to Darwin wharf and two nuns were there: Sister Benedicta and another one, and myself and the captain of the boat, Don or something. I went across to Gurindin and got off at the Gurindin wharf. I met one yeller-feller, Jack. He knows a little bit of my language and I did like him too much because he knows my language. I couldn't speak even one word of English.

I went up to dormitory; that's where Rrangura was staying. I didn't know him. He was sleeping beside me. But he couldn't talk to me because we didn't know each other, see! We went to the dining room that day. We had porridge and milk. I didn't have porridge before, but I had it in Darwin Hospital. I had an egg. Then Lambu came along and this other bloke whose name was Paddy. Billhembu and Sea Water came along, and Lipa Lipa and Marrala and they had to introduce me to Rrangura, and then I knew him: but I couldn't speak to him before. And then I'm allowed to follow him around to the school and dining-room, because he knew better that place. I was a bit worried, you know, because I wanted to come back here to Elcho Island.

It took me a long time to know everyone there and to get to like them. Rrangura was in the school, with Lambu and Ronnie and Michael and Joey and Dawson and Victor and Maurice and Leslie and Sweeney. Sister was teaching us: I don't know his name but he was a good teacher. I didn't know too much English but I learned. I was there at Gurindin only for two months, and then at East Arm. I had tablets for burundiya, and bandages

as well. I was getting better a little bit because I could see it. My sores were getting smaller and smaller. I was feeling happy. And then two years went past and I wanted to stay there. I didn't worry for my father any more. I forgot about him. I got used to the people over there. I used to go to school in the morning for half a day and then work in the afternoon at the hospital. I worked with Fred and Terry and even Rrangura, and then another year went by.

They took me over to the clinic, doing the feet and hands and giving out burundiya tablets every morning, and iron and calcium tablet with burundiya tablets. Every morning I used to work there at the clinic with the sisters and the clinic boys, Ray and Oscar, who came after me, and Matches. Mother Marion was the boss nun and before her, Mother Benedicta. She was the toughest when we do wrong things, like smokes and so on. We were bad—we knew we were bad at East Arm. They called East Arm 'Mosquito-early' because them mosquitoes came too early in the morning.

Yeah! I worked there from 1956, 1957, 1958, 1959, 1960, 1961 and 1962. I went away in 1963. You [Dr Hargrave] sent me home in 1963. Marrku [perhaps] you thought I was better. I thought myself it was because me and Terry had an argument and I didn't want to work in the hospital any more. Me and Terry had an argument about plasters. He wanted me to put plaster on Joey and I said, 'I'm too busy and you doing nothing—you can do that.' I told him, and he went to Mother and told her, and Mother and two sisters came around and I said, 'I'm too busy and I can't do this and I'm going to leave you now. I'll go somewhere else to work.'

So I'm going to Sonny Bennett and I worked there with Sonny Bennett and then I didn't stay long. I didn't work long enough with Sonny, only two months. You sent me back to the Mission. It was four months before I found work—just hunting. I had presents from the school. I had rations—morning, dinnertime, suppertime—flour, syrup, sugar and fish. I went for fish with a fishing line.

Then four months went by. I went to

Bapa Sheppie and ask him for a job and he give me a job making roads from Mission to the other side, a place called Galawarra. It took us four months with axe and shovel and mattocks. I finish from there and I went away to Yirrkala on the canoe, a real big canoe belong to my grandfather, to Yirrkala. Darawa [plenty] shark and porpoise and dugong and stingrays and turtles. We went to Mata Mata and we couldn't go any further because we were heading against the wind. It was September. We had to stay there for three weeks at a place called Wurwala [Bluna]. We put sail on, a square one, Macassar rig, and from Wurwala no stops till we got to Melville Bay. Just one day—it's not far—we stopped about half past five. We camped at Waritjapa [King's Village] and we left the canoe now. It is Wallaby Beach and you can still camp there. It is a special place for Rumbul. He is Yirritja; he's a Gumatj. I'm Dhuwa: I'm Galpu. Kupapuingu is Yirritja. Liyagawumirri is Dhuwa and Liyagalawumirri is Dhuwa. We camped at Wallaby Beach and we had to wait for the moon to come up and the tide to go down. We left the camp here.

We walked from Wallaby Beach all night, right round, the long way round. From Wallaby Beach we went across the creek to a place called Lumua; from there right up to Tarluru, another creek there. From there we crossed to Garalatami where the town is, called Town Beach now. From there we went right up to Bukulungai—Rainbow Cliff today—and from there to Djarwuluku Hills; that place is called Dreaming Head today. From there to Yirrkala now. From Yarmunna we could see the houses. Daybreaking we didn't light fire. First time I went to Yirrkala. Nobody didn't know me there—not even my sister or my grandma didn't know me.

So I went there. My uncle, he came over and shook hands with me and the other young boys. There were about eleven of us. He told us to follow him. My mother's brother he was. So I went there to my uncle's place. He didn't know me. So I sat down to breakfast—damper and tea, bayngu [nothing] meat. Darawa [plenty] meat at Mata Mata—turtle and dugong. No hunting at Yirrkala because they had

no canoe. I stayed there and some people were asking about me: 'Who's he? Where does he come from?' One of my stepbrothers said, 'This is Yawirongga.' And they thought I was still over at Gurindin.

You know how they do silly things when they see you for the first time—cry over you and hit their head with a stick, Yolngu way. I stayed there for one year, just a holiday. I chased up the mielk [girls]; only caught one. I haven't got that one now; she's not married to anyone. She's still after me; she works at the office at Yirrkala. She still wants me; I want her. What do you think? I think I'll get her. She's promised to some other fellow. She's my uncle's daughter. I have to pay for the mielk [girl]. Last time when we ran off—last month that was—they said, 'You'll have to give us $300.' Where the hell I could get that much money? One of my friend said, 'These two women, they are not boat or motorcar: they're human beings.' One of the police-trackers said that. That mielk is a different one. That one I had at East Arm is from here. She's all right, but her father don't want me to marry her because she belongs to the other tribe; she is Dalwangu. My father told me I've got to go and marry to my mother's tribe: Gumatj.

The girl, the one who's after me, she's promised to Flock of Parrots, you know, who was at East Arm. I'm not going to pay him but I'm going to pay the mother of the girl. That's the one I took before. The one I took over to East Arm. She's coming back. They agree with me because she's got my child. He's about two years old. I've had three 'wives' but that other one: I told her not to come back because she and that other girl that I'm after, they fight over me and I didn't like it. They're both at Yirrkala. Where can I find all this money?

Five years ago, maybe, I was sniffing that petrol. I don't know why: maybe just for fun. And this money I used to get, I used to work little bit harder but some people got more than me, you know. We were round here making roads. I was trying to get something else. And then I thought, 'Ah! No use working and getting little bit of money and others getting more than me. No use working. I'll have to do something. Pinch some money: go to schoolhouse and pinch some money.' Then I sent some of the boys to Bapa Sheppie's place; pinched some money from there. I sent some of the boys—pinch some more. I was the head. I wanted more money; so I had friends and I had some boys, you know, to do nothing but steal everything.

I didn't know what I was going to do. I just wanted money and I pinched this boat here, the big one, Djupari. I went to Marchinba on this boat. It was Friday night and people down here were having ceremony: a bunggul to make young man, you know. It was about half past seven. I went down to the beach, poured some petrol in the fruit tin, soaked some rags and then sniffed until I was, you know, feel funny up on my head. I went down, pulled a dinghy. I had three boys with me: Lambul, Lipal Lipa and Marrayala. We went down there and hopped board the Djupari.

I told them to pull the anchor and start the engine. It has tucker and fish and syrup and sugar; everything in it. Some of the fishermen forgot to take it ashore. So I started the engine and off I went—down the point round there to Wessel Islands to Marchinba. There were some boys over there. They were there for three months for the same thing—sniffing petrol, you know! They were sad to come back home. I went there and my brother went over to Rarakala—that's another island—he went there and he asked me if I wanted to come back because I was sore on my knee and I said, 'Yes, I'll go there,' and I told the boys I'll be back Saturday. 'With what?' they said. I said 'I'm going to take one of the boats'.

I went to Rarakala and I got there at half past five in the morning and they were ready to go across from Rarakala to another island called Djilkari. They saw the boat and they saw me come round the point and they knew it was me. And I went there and told them to come aboard and I said, 'Come on everybody, come on board.' I told them, even the old man was there, old Galatharra—he used to look after the boys, the petrol sniffers—me and Mangata, my father's brother. I told them to come aboard and everything and they asked: 'Where

you're going to take us? To Marchinba?' But I told them, 'No, we're going back home to the Mission'. Oh, yes. We short of tobacco and everything. We got trousers all torn up. Some of them have to wear naga [loin cloth].

It was Saturday. We anchored here about half past seven. Everybody came down to the beach there, even Balanda. The fisherman, you know he was the boss, Bunggawa—his name was Merv Anderson—Daynbirri we used to call him. 'Hello Skipper', he said to me and I said, 'Hello.' 'How's the boat?' he said. 'Oh, it's in good order, everything's OK', I said. 'What about the ngata [food]?' 'Oh', I said, 'finished it up; I was hungry'.

All right; then next day they told me to make a road from there to there. I was with the boys that came back with me making them roads for nothing, just for tucker, because I took the boat. I was doing that for a month, two months. Then came the police. They asked me, 'Why did you take it? Where did you take it? Did you pinch anything else from the boat?' I said, 'No, I didn't take nothing; it's all there'.

They asked me to go over to Darwin for the court. Well I was there for three months, you know, that time. I was in Fannie Bay Gaol: good place, good food, plenty food, and wireless. And then I went to the burundiya clinic, then you came along and picked me up. I said, 'I won't get drunk again', but I got drunk and then you told me to go away, but I'll forgive you for that!—I broke my promise. The next day on Saturday you told Jack Scrymgour to take us over to Bagot, so he did. I stayed there in Bagot for four weeks: no jobs, no ngata [food].

My father sent me some money; it was five dollars or seven dollars and then I had some nata and then the Warrawi came along. Red Sky was the captain. I went up to the Mission Office at Darwin. I asked Wawa David Stewart if he can put me on the Warrawi.

So Wawa Stewart said, 'Go down and see Captain Red Sky'. So I went down to the wharf in Darwin and I asked Red Sky and he said, 'You can come along', and he asked me if I had any money and then Wawa Stewart told Red Sky, 'He can make up for that—he can work along with you while he is going back. He can do a bit of work on the boat'. And so I did. I came back from Darwin on the Warrawi. We sailed on Tuesday. We left from Darwin about half past eight in the morning and we anchored in Barnin—near Cape Don.

From there next morning we sailed and we anchored in Goulburn Island. We went right past Croker Island and from Goulburn Island right up to Sandy Island. We had dinner there and we anchored there. We had oysters and crayfish and in the afternoon we sailed across to Maningrida. It was Friday. We anchored at Maningrida about half past five. We went ashore to see the pictures. We stayed overnight there. Next morning we sailed again. From there, right up to Milingimbi, on Sunday. The tide was low, you know. We didn't have time to unload the cargo. So next morning, Monday, we started unloading the cargo. About half past ten we left Milingimbi. From Milingimbi we anchored here about five o'clock at Elcho. We unloaded some cargo, only for one day, and next day we left for Yirrkala, right up to Melville Bay.

We came back here to the Mission, then I got a job on the hygiene. I worked here for about one year though. I was going straight until some blokes came from Mata Mata and they kept saying, 'What about this petrol?' So I started again, sniffing petrol. From there I went to breaking into the school. No petrol in the school but I had some in the pannikin. The petrol makes me do anything, silly things, sometimes, we know. I broke in and pinched some money in the school. I can't remember how much but I remember I had $250, and I gave some away to the other boys who were with me. I couldn't count it because it was dark, you know; and one four gallon drum of sugar [petrol]. I went down to the cemetery and I hid it there; covered it up with leaves and then every night we used to go out with pannikin each and get sugar from the tin. We had teas.

Then one day Wawa Kevin Davis—he was the school teacher—he went up to the school and he was looking for the sugar. And I don't know how he knew it

was me and he went down to my father and he said, 'Where's Yawirongga?' And my father said, 'He's inside sleeping'. He came along and knocked on the door and I woke up and he said, 'Where's my sugar?' And I said, 'I don't know where is your sugar'. And he said, 'Is that true?' And well, I couldn't help so I had to tell lie.

And then I thought, I'll just have to tell him. He had turned around, so I called him back: 'Wawa, I got your sugar'. 'And where my money is?' And I stand still for a moment and I gave him back his money—about $200. When I gave him the money, well I thought he was satisfied with the money but he went to the Superintendent up here and asked him to ring up for the police. So he rang up for the police.

We went to Darwin, all went to Darwin by aeroplane, by charter. Landed on Gunbalanya [Oenpelli], filled up some petrol and from there we flew right on to Darwin, straight into the monkey-house [police station]. Next morning we went to court and we had one Balanda from Welfare. I don't know what his name; well, he was with us and we were free, but I think we should really be fined. I think he gave us some piece of paper with money on it; well, he gave us a fortnight for us to pay, but no job. We went all over looking for a job, even went to Bagot to Davis Daniels, and then I went back to gaol for seven days because I couldn't pay—no djama [work] and then I went to East Arm.

I was drunk. I went to the clinic in Darwin and I ask one of the yapas [Sisters] there. I was short of money and I wanted to come back to the Mission. She said, 'All right, you can go on Friday'. Well I stayed here for a month, and then I didn't want to stay here. I went to Yirrkala, and then I was no good. Went to Wallaby Beach. I was drinking there then—VB [Victoria Bitter]—darawa [lots] cartons every day. I was drinking; I was happy. I was looking for a place to camp. I walked around; I couldn't find nothing to cover myself. It was cold weather, so I went up to ask some Balanda for matches. I asked one man there and he gave me a box of matches. I went down to the beach and gathered fire woods and I lit the fire and I went to sleep. I was sleeping all right—good way—during the night until about daybreak!

I turned over and put my left knee beside the fire and I couldn't feel it because of the burundiya. It must have been there for some time. From that day I had this sore for nearly one year. Plenty times tried to fix it. I had this sore on my knee from last year, but I was always running away—mielk [girl] and nanidji [liquor] problems—all that. I went back to East Arm and then you did this job properly and I stayed in bed because I had the mielk with me. Before I had this bandage around my knee and every time I walked the bandage rubbed and I didn't know; I couldn't feel it—this burundiya. I had this skin graft and you turned this knee over. I'm going straight now.

I encountered Yawirongga again at the Mission three years after he told Dr Hargrave this story. He was walking down the cliff-top road, airily swinging a machete, accompanied by a short, plump, happy-looking wife carrying the baby. He was walking quite comfortably. He wore no bandages and the cavernous ulcer I had seen on his knee, with widespread loss of surrounding skin, had disappeared entirely. This astonished me because I remembered it at its worst, with straw stuffed behind the knee cap. Now, after Dr Hargrave's skin grafts, it was whole; and so was Yawirongga. He seemed domesticated and settled, recovered from leprosy, and without any air of stigma. He had a bit of the vagrant about him, resisting local assimilation, with an itinerant way of life. At heart, a wanderer.

He was partial to sniffing petrol and drinking grog but without shame. He was more itinerant than outcast, as well as an optimist. The chief effects of his leprosy, and the long treatment away from home, have been to leave him loosely attached, perhaps leading a gypsy's life, inclined to the excitement of the prevailing intoxicants. He has given us his story to help us understand what leprosy does to a man's life.

I began by saying that leprosy was not one malaise but two: a disease and a stigma. I might have said four: disease, stigma, disownment and pay-back. Yawirongga's particular blessing is his unawareness of stigma and pay-back, although his life reflects some rootlessness and wandering. All that he suffers from is leprosy, and Dr Hargrave helped him overcome it. What we have to appraise, in his case, is his seeming disregard of the social factors that often unite to make this disease the worst of all, bearing the curses of stigma and pay-back. This has something to do with innate happiness and tough-mindedness, though I hardly know where those qualities come from. I wish I did. And he has travelled Arnhem Land more than most of his kind.

1 Hargrave, J (1970) *Leprosy in Northern Territory Aborigines* Australian Department of Health Canberra.

APHRODISIACS for CHINA

For centuries before any Europeans mad
Macassans from Celebes voyaged along
the magical needs of wealthy Chinese
Arnhem Land is the sea cucumber or se
dweller of those shallow tepid waters of
dine on it, if they can find nothing better
is worthless to them. Yet it once found a
It became the subject of a dream.

The Chinese dreamed that it was a panacea for their ills, and this dream sent Indonesian fishermen in their thousands to these territorial waters to gather it for the Chinese market. They called it trepang, or beche-de-mer. Yolngu tell me that eating trepang can affect your mind strangely so that you feel unreal and become delirious—if you survive the vomiting and diarrhoea. The exotic disease from which you would suffer if you chanced to eat trepang might be called holothurian intoxication, for that is the name of the toxic glucoside this animal harbours. This is a saponin, a class of substance occurring naturally and

an impact on the people and the shores of Arnhem Land,
hat coastline, harvesting a little animal intended to meet
The most prolific and most disregarded animal in
lug. Either name describes it well enough. It is a bottom
he territorial seas of Northern Australia. Some turtles may
o eat. Man and fish pass it by without a second glance. It
place, not an unimportant place, in the course of history.

able to form a lather. Mixtures of saponins are used in detergents and as the foam producer in fire extinguishers. Some saponins are toxic, like the holothurian of our humble trepang.

If it is poisonous, what made the Chinese nation go into such raptures about trepang? For centuries Chinese merchants engaged caravels to go to the unknown South Land to garner it by the tonne from those shores and take it to Timor, whence their own junks sailed it home to the local markets to sell for food and for medicine. They called it sea-ginseng and they prized it as much as the horticultural variety of ginseng, *Panax schinseng*, the palmate plant of East Asia whose root is prized by the vast population as a panacea. It carries little charisma in the non-Asian world. Herbal shops in Australia have a small turnover, a popular brand being Blackmore's Ginseng, produced by laboratories in Auckland, New Zealand. It is more cautiously advertised on the bottle as 'systemic tonic'.

Trepang, when boiled, dried and smoked for use in soups or braised in a wok with vegetables, becomes an acceptable food free from poison. It is said to bring out the flavour of other foods but its popularity is increased by its reputation as a nervous stimulant and aphrodisiac. It came into widespread use in China in the late Ming period, around the same time as other exotic foods such as birds' nests and sharks' fins. Trepang achieved no popularity among Westerners either as food or medicine; as for Aborigines, they passed it by for culinary use, because it needs boiling, a process not possible for them.

Trade from Australia to China was longstanding before the first export cargo sailed from Sydney Town for England. Australia's first modern industry was trepang. The most informative book on the history of this subject is probably *The Voyage to Marege* by C C Macknight.[1] Marege was the name given by sailors from Macassar to this part of Northern Australia. Macassar is now called Ujung Pandang, in Indonesia's Sulawesi.[2]

During the centuries of trade—prohibited by the Commonwealth of Australia after Federation in 1901—the Macassan visitors imparted many aspects of their culture to Aborigines living in northern Australia. The only other contacts were passing visits by the Portuguese, Dutch and English in the ships of the navigator-explorers.

Few people now inhabit this coastline, and fewer still know those who do. The Arafura Sea, which is a wide plain only inundated since the last Ice Age, lies between the Australian coast in the south, the island of Timor of the Republic of Indonesia in the west, and the Indonesian territory of Irian Jaya in the north. It is one of the seas of the world least navigated or traversed, especially today. It is a well-defended stronghold of mosquitoes against humans. However, it was not always so desolate.

We have seen that for three centuries before the twentieth, swaying fleets of caravels ploughed down from Celebes, to Timor and then to New Holland, propelled by the north-west monsoons, seeking the treasure of these shallow waters. We have heard that the prize was trepang, a prize which is now as despised as its own habitat. Notwithstanding its present obscurity we should pause to regard its former fame, for nothing will give us a better sense of the exotic character of these shores, the stirring events they generated, and the modern dramas which they set in train.

Naturalists place trepang in the phylum of echinoderms, class of holothurians. It frequents the intertidal zone of the Australian coast of

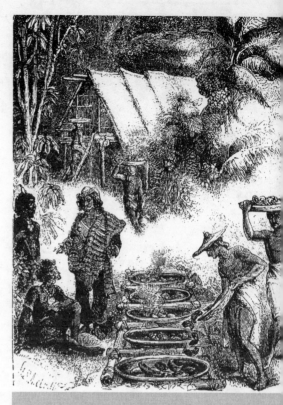

Macassans at Victoria, Port Essington, in 1845, by H S Melville.

the Arafura Sea, and somewhat deeper. For so sluggish an animal it breeds prolifically. It feeds with tentacles around the mouth, taking in algae, detritus and sand. It probably also feeds through the tentacles on its body, which trap tiny creatures in the mucus on each tentacle. When it is attacked it has a surprising response: it expels a sticky mass of tubules in spurts from its anus; sometimes it throws out other internal organs and dies. These jets of turbid fluid can injure the skin or eyes of the attacker.

Although the trepang resembles a cucumber in shape, to the Chinese eye of faith and hope it resembled the erect male organ—somewhat more grand than most—and its propensity to expel turbid fluid when aroused added to this fantasy. These orgasmic death throes (folklore would have us

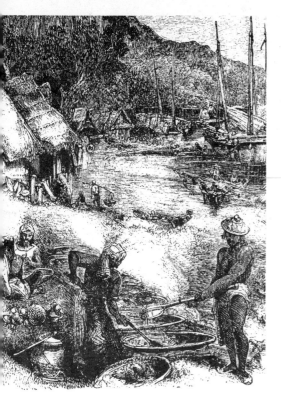

believe that murderers at the cross-tree also climax sexually at the end of the fourteen-foot drop from the tree with a halter around their neck) recommended trepang to the Chinese, but not only as a result of the theory of sympathetic magic. The Chinese name for trepang is *hai-sen*, meaning sea-ginseng, which should tell us something. Toxicological study shows that the toxic saponin holothurian, contained in the tissues of trepang, causes interesting effects in laboratory animals. We know little or nothing of its toxicity to humans, save that it affects the nervous system. For this reason the Macassan fishermen boiled it several times in water, which they changed daily, or claimed they did: supervision of workers is not always dependable. Without a doubt some consignments of trepang affected the nervous system.

How did this humble echinoderm come to captivate the gourmets of China? It was not by virtue of any piquancy as an article of the diet; even less by virtue of nutritional value. Presumably it filled a need generated by the theoretical considerations of the patrimonial Chinese medicine. Under that system of scholarship the vital substances of yin and yang possess a polarity of effect. Yin is female and negative, inducing hypostates and cold diseases; yang is male and positive, inducing hyperstates and hot diseases like fevers. The axiom is that yang creates yin; yang destroys yin. Yin and yang mutually support and sustain. They must be in harmony or equally strong for normal balance in the body. The solid organs—heart, lungs, kidney and spleen—are all yin and energy storers; the hollow organs—bowel, gall-bladder and the triple warmer, the pleural, abdominal and pelvic cavities—are all yang and energy dischargers. The life energy, chi, circulates through the body along meridians, amenable to influence at some thousand or more tender points, available for insertion of needles by acupuncture and moxibustion.

The humble trepang thus found itself exalted by a poetic metaphor; it became a much sought-after item of diet as a yang producer. With its phallic shape it became a symbol of virility and potency; at length an aphrodisiac of renown. It was imported in vast quantities. The Macassan fishermen, ever attuned to the Chinese need for sympathetic magic, and their own need for profit, came to the Arnhem Land coast each summer and procured it, hundreds of piculs of it, for the Chinese consumer. But the local Yolngu, who subsist by the providence of nature in this region, neglected the trepang. They would not take the trouble to harvest it from the

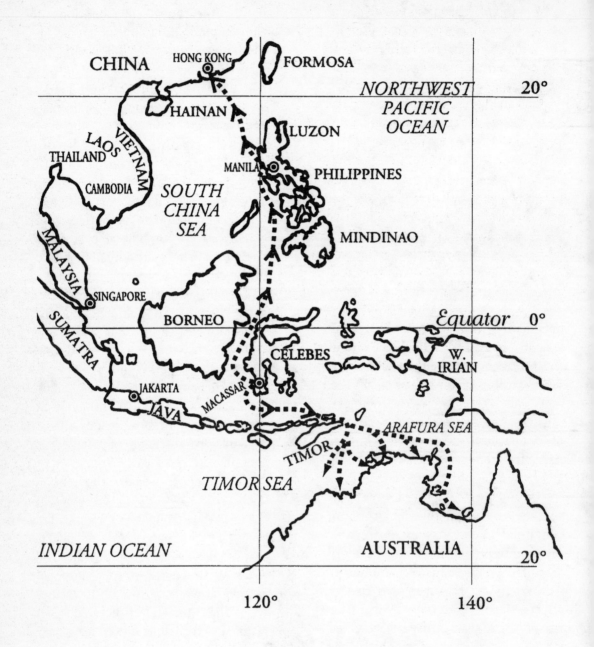

The route taken by trepang traders in the Far East during the seventeenth,
eighteenth and nineteenth centuries.

floor of their own sea even if they were starving. It was poisonous. And they had no need of aphrodisiacs—a need that perhaps arises from reading too many learned scrolls, written by Buddhist holy men in monastic cells.

The European latecomers to the South Land are not particularly aware of this Asian connection, being commonly instructed that the outside world's contact with Australia began with Captain James Cook. But if they were, they might see some irony in the historical fact that this country which came to be called Australia had for its first trade a valueless commodity whose esteem rested on a popular delusion, an induced belief of some gullible masses. But these Arnhem Landers know better: they welcomed some Macassan trepang fishermen, and hurled their spears at others.

These visitors now brought a new significance to the north-west monsoon as the wind that brought gifts from over the shoulder of the world— gifts they coveted. These visitors in their caravels merely removed trepang and pearl shell, items too plentiful to be of value, and in return they brought priceless treasures—tobacco, fermented liquor and various tools of iron. With an iron axe, a man can hew a dugout canoe, seaworthy in deep water, capable of reaching the most remote of the thirty-four islands. With an iron spear-head, he can prevail in a dispute and become the master. And with Dutch gin, in glass or pottery vessels, he can utterly transcend the trials and tribulations of daily life. The first Australians had not discovered the miracle of fermented liquor, not because they had no grain, but because they had no vats to ferment it in and no pottery to store it in. A good cask needs strong staves and iron bands.

The thirty-four islands where these events took place lie in the Arafura Sea between 11 degrees and 12 degrees of south latitude, and 136 degrees and 138 degrees of west longitude. The Malay Road, traditional roadstead of the trepang fishers from the north, separates the most southerly line of these islands from the mainland of Australia. The introduction of dugout canoe technology permitted Arnhem Landers, these Yolngu (a vernacular name for 'our people') to settle these offshore islands. By their new skill and daring they became deep-water sailors. They took the thirty-four islands as their territory. From any one of these islands you can see the next or most adjacent islands if you peer from the highest vantage point, and so on until you have the thirty-four on your mental chart.

As seafarers, Aboriginal deep-water sailors evolved a distinctive way of living in the world and of looking at it. Few of us know much about it as it has not been the subject of much study. Of those who know it, some consider that way of life unique; some, beautiful; but some, too dangerous and fragile to survive. Indeed it came to pass, with the foreclosure of the trepang harvest by the infant Australian Commonwealth in the early years of the twentieth century, that the Malay Road became only a memory. It is important to be clear that it was white and not black Australians who called a halt to the annual visits of the Macassan trepang fleets, by imposing an impossible tax on them.

The main concern in the mind of the infant Federation of Australia was to check an anticipated Chinese inundation of the dimensions that charac-

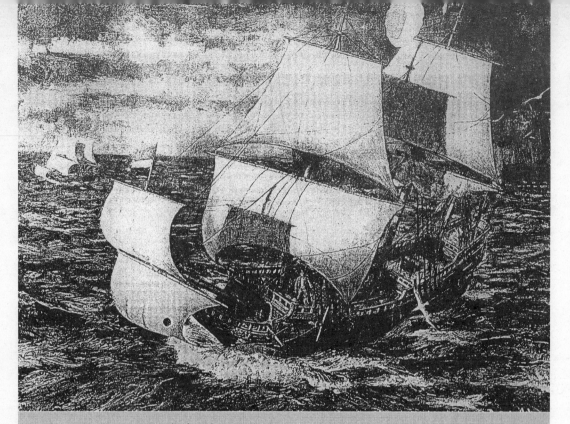

Arnhem Land was named after the Dutch ship *Arnhem* sent out in 1623 by the Governor of the West Indies to explore the land to the south. When the ship reached what is now Cape York Peninsula it was blown right across the gulf where the crew discovered new coast on the other side. To this land they gave the name of their ship, the Arnhem.[3] (Painting by Dennis Adams.)

terized the gold rushes not long before. But it also closed the era of trade with the Celebes, a trade to which Yolngu had adjusted their lifestyle. The dugout canoe was the craft that enabled them to colonize large offshore islands, like Groote Eylandt in the Gulf of Carpentaria and the Wessel Islands in the Arafura Sea. Then followed the demise of the dugout canoe, and with that, the decline and fall of the thirty-four-island empire. Many of the islanders died—or self-annihilated. Some re-treated from the outlying islands to the mainland. Some burned their boats literally and ceremoniously, not merely metaphorically. I have seen it done. But of those who were left, all kept their distinctive visions of the thirty-four islands in their mind's eye ... 'For oft, when on my couch I lie ... They flash upon that inward eye ... In public, they paid homage to the well-known heroes of the mainland clans, as was required. In private they planned to return to their islands when the time was ripe. They were saltwater people: they could not pros-per until the day that they should return to the saltwater.

The people remembered the great days of trepang, even if they never appreciated trepang itself. This fasci-nating history is well set down in C C Macknight's *The Voyage to Marege*. But the most exciting account of trepang history is bound to be the first. It comes from Matthew Flinders' own ship's log, ultimately printed as *A*

Voyage to Terra Australis,[4] published in two volumes and atlas in 1814 in London. Matthew Flinders sailed on that voyage for the purpose of charting the coastline of this vast country in the years 1801, 1802 and 1803, in His Majesty's sloop *Investigator*. Flinders was very unlucky on his trip home to England. At that time England was at war with France, led by the Emperor Napoleon. Flinders called at Mauritius, the French colony in the Indian Ocean, expecting to get water and supplies. Instead, he was imprisoned by the French governor of that island for six and a half years. It ruined his life and his health. When he finally got home to London he was no hero, no hero at all! He had played no part in the war in which England had vanquished Napoleon, who had tried to spread the French Empire all over Europe. The Emperor Napoleon was overcome and was exiled to a small island in the South Atlantic Ocean, just as Flinders was imprisoned on a small island in the Indian Ocean.

In the following account, the reader should bear in mind that when Captain Flinders encountered the Malays he and probably most of his crew were affected by scurvy. The prophylaxis advocated by Dr James Lind[5] had not yet been satisfactorily adopted by the Royal Navy, and scurvy remained the scourge of long sea voyagers. And HM sloop *Investigator* was a scurvy ship, rotten with shipworm. So here, with the deepest of respect, is what Flinders recorded in his log. It tells us more about the trepang than we should ever know about this unlikely food of delusion and wish fulfilment. I hope you find it as exciting as I do.

After clearing the narrow passage between Cape Wilberforce and Bromby's Isles, we followed the main coast to the S.W.; having on the starboard hand some high and large islands, which closed in towards the coast ahead so as to make it doubtful whether there were any passage between them. Under the nearest island was perceived a canoe full of men; and in a sort of roadstead, at the south end of the same island, there were six vessels covered over like hulks, as if laid up for the bad season. Our conjectures were various as to who those people could be, and what their business here; but we had little doubt of their being the same, whose traces had been found so abundantly in the Gulph. I had inclined to the opinion that these traces had been left by Chinese, and the report of the natives in Caledon Bay that they had fire arms, strengthened the supposition; and combining this with the appearance of the vessels, I set them down for piratical Ladrones who secreted themselves here from pursuit, and issued out as the season permitted, or prey invited them. Impressed with this idea, we tacked to work up for the road; and our pendant and ensign being hoisted, each of them hung out a small white flag. On approaching, I sent Lieutenant Flinders in an armed boat, to learn who they were; and soon afterward we came to an anchor in 12 fathoms, within musket shot; having a spring on the cable, and all hands at quarters.

Every motion in the whale boat, and in the vessel alongside which she was lying, was closely watched with our glasses, but all seemed to pass quietly; and on the return of Lieutenant Flinders, we learned that they were prows from Macassar, and the six Malay commanders shortly afterwards came on board in a canoe. It happened fortunately that my cook was a Malay, and through his means I was able to communicate with them. The chief of the six prows was a short, elderly man, named Pobassoo; he said there were upon the coast, in different division, sixty prows, and that Salloo was the commander in chief. These people were Mahometans, and on looking into the launch, expressed great horror to see hogs there; nevertheless they had no objection to port wine, and even requested a bottle to carry away with them at sunset.

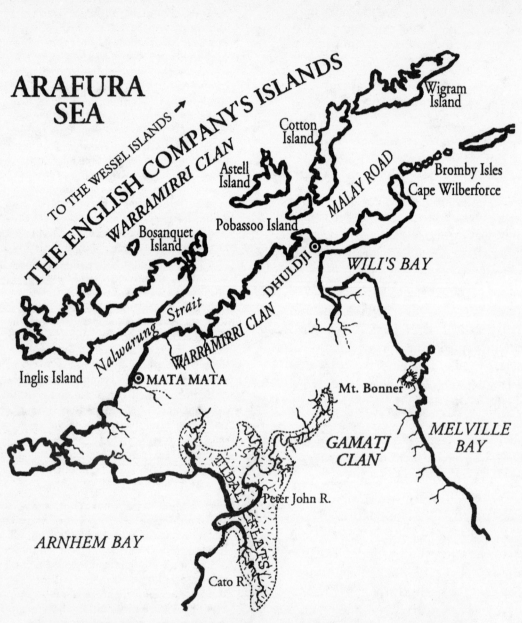

ARAFURA
SEA

TO THE WESSEL ISLANDS →

THE ENGLISH COMPANY'S ISLANDS

WARRAMIRRI CLAN

Wigram
Island

Cotton
Island

Astell
Island

Bosanquet
Island

Pobassoo Island

MALAY ROAD

Bromby Isles
Cape Wilberforce

DHULDJI

WILI'S BAY

Nalwarung Strait

WARRAMIRRI CLAN

Inglis Island

⊚ MATA MATA

Mt. Bonner

MELVILLE
BAY

GAMATJ
CLAN

TIDAL FLATS

Peter John R.

ARNHEM BAY

Cato R.

WARRAMIRRI HOMELANDS

The weather continued squally all night, with frequent heavy rain, and the wind blew strong; but coming off the islands, the ship rode easily. In the morning, I went on board Pobassoo's vessel, with two of the gentlemen and my interpreter, to make further inquiries; and afterwards the six chiefs came to the Investigator, and several canoes were alongside for the purpose of barter. Before noon, five other prows steered into the road from the S.W., anchoring near the former six; and we had more people about the ship that I chose to admit on board, for each of them wore a short dagger or cress by his side. My people were under arms, and the guns were exercised and a shot fired at the request of the chiefs; in the evening they all retired quietly, but our guns were kept ready and half the people at quarters all night. The weather was very rainy; and towards morning, much noise was heard amongst the prows. At daylight they got under sail, and steered through the narrow passage between Cape Wilberforce and Bromby's Isles, by which we had come; and afterwards directed their course south-eastward into the Gulph of Carpentaria.

My desire to learn everything concerning these people, and the strict look-out which it had been necessary to keep upon them, prevented me attending to any other business during their stay. According to Pobassoo, from whom my information was principally obtained, sixty prows belonging to the Rajah of Boni, and carrying one thousand men, had left Macassar with the north-west monsoon, two months before, upon an expedition to this coast; and the fleet was then lying in different places to the westward, five or six together, Pobassoo's division being the foremost. These prows seemed to be about twenty-five tons, and to have twenty or twenty-five men in each; that of Pobassoo carried two small brass guns, obtained from the Dutch, but the others had only muskets; besides which, every Malay wears a cress or dagger, either secretly or openly. I inquired after bows and arrows, and the ippo poison, but they had none of them; and it was with difficulty they could understand what was meant by the ippo.

The object of their expedition was a certain marine animal, called trepang. Of this they gave me two dried specimens; and it proved to be the bêche-de-mer, or sea cucumber which we had first seen on the reefs of the East Coast, and had afterwards hauled on shore so plentifully with the seine, especially in Caledon Bay. They get the trepang by diving in from 3 to 8 fathoms water; and where it is abundant, a man will bring up eight or ten at a time. The mode of preserving it is this: the animal is split down one side, boiled, and pressed with a weight of stones; then stretched open by slips of bamboo, dried in the sun, and afterwards in smoke, when it is fit to be put away in bags, but requires frequent exposure to the sun. A thousand trepang make a picol, of about 125 Dutch pounds; and one hundred picols are a cargo for a prow. It is carried to Timor, and sold to the Chinese, who meet them there; and when all the prows are assembled, the fleet returns to Macassar. By Timor, seemed to be meant Timor-laoet; for when I inquired concerning the English, Dutch, and Portuguese there, Pobassoo knew nothing of them: he had heard of Coepang, a Dutch settlement, but said it was upon another island.

Pobassoo had made six or seven voyages from Macassar to this coast, within the preceding twenty years, and he was one of the first who came; but had never seen any ship here before. This road was the first rendezvous for his division, to take in water previously to going into the Gulph. One of their prows had been lost the year before, and much inquiry was made concerning the pieces of wreck we had seen; and a canoe's rudder being produced it was recognised as having belonged to her. They sometimes had skirmishes with the native inhabitants of the coast; Pobassoo himself had been formerly speared in the knee, and a man had been slightly wounded since their arrival in this road: they cautioned us much to beware of the natives.

My numberless questions were answered patiently, and with apparent sincerity; Pobassoo even stopped one day longer at my desire, than he had intended, for the north-west monsoon, he said, would not blow quite a month longer, and he was rather late. I rewarded his trouble and that of his companions with several presents, principally iron tools, which they seemed anxious to possess; and he begged of me an English jack, which he afterwards carried at the head of his squadron. He also expressed a desire for a letter, to show to any other ship he might meet; and I accordingly wrote him a note to Captain Baudin, whom it seemed probable he might encounter in the Gulph, either going or returning.

From the 19th to the 22nd, the weather was frequently rainy, with thunder and lightning; and the wind blew strong in squalls, generally between the north and west, and made it unsafe to move the ship. During these days, the botanical gentlemen overran the two islands which form Malay Road; and I made a boat excursion to Astell's, and another to the north end of Cotton's Island, to sound and take bearings for the survey. In the latter excursion, three black children were perceived on the north-east beach; and on walking that way we saw two bark huts, and an elderly man was sitting under a tree, near them. He smiled on finding himself discovered, and went behind a bush, when a confused noise was heard of women and children making off into the wood; the man also retreated up the hill, and our friendly signs were ineffectual to stop him. In one of the huts was a net bag, containing some pieces of gum, bone, and a broken spike nail; and against a neighbouring bush were standing three spears, one of which had a number of barbs, and had been wrought with some ingenuity. This I took away; but the rest of the arms, with the utensils and furniture of the huts, consisting of the foresaid net bag and a shell to drink out of, were left as we found them, with the addition of a hatchet and pocket handkerchief.

The upper surfaces of these islands are barren; but in the valleys, down which ran streams of water at this time, there is a tolerable soil. One of these valleys, at the south end of Cotton's Island, might be made a delightful situation to a college of monks, who could bear the heat of the climate, and were impenetrable to the stings of musketoes. Here grew the wild nutmeg, in abundance, the fig

which bears its fruit on the stem, two species of palm, and a tree whose bark is in common use in the East for making ropes; besides a variety of others, whose tops were overspread with creeping vines, forming a shade to the stream underneath. But this apparently delightful retreat afforded anything rather than coolness and tranquillity: the heat was suffocating, and the musketoes admitted not of a moment's repose.

Upon Pobassoo's Island, near the stream of water at the back of the beach, Mr Good, the gardener, planted four of the cocoa nuts procured from the Malays; and also some remnants of potatoes which were found in the ship.

We saw no other stone on the low shores than iron ore, similar to that found in the upper part of Melville Bay, and on Point Middle in Caledon Bay; and it seems probable that iron runs through the space of country comprehended between the heads of the three bays, although the exterior shores and the hills be either granitic, argillaceous, or of sand stone. The flat country where the iron ore is found, seems to afford a good soil, well-clothed with grass and wood, much superior to that where granite or sand stone prevails; this I judge from what was seen near the heads of the bays, for our excursions inland were necessarily very confined, and for myself, I did not quit the water side at Arnhem Bay, being disabled by scorbutic ulcers on my feet.

Coming back from poor Captain Flinders, disabled by scorbutic sores, to the Yolngu and their disregard for the prize that the Chinese crossed half a world to win, Yolngu may not gather it but they do not entirely despise it. They know its place. The trepang is called *warripa* in Warramirri dialect and is of the Yirritja moiety, part of the household of that irrepressible trickster god, Marryalyan.[6] Under Marryalyan, warripa has a sexual energy to impart for those who know.

My brother Stingray Spine described it in this way.

There are several foods which keep up your sexual energy and lubricate sexual movement. All fish will do it, especially the dugong, and the trepang above all. And get some heart of palm if you can!

When I was a diver for trepang on Fred Gray's boat we would save some trepang after a big dive. This was in 1936, on board the Ortili. He sold it to the Chinese in Darwin, and to a dealer on Thursday Island. Some of the trepang we took in Caledon Bay, the rest in Arnhem Bay. Well, when Fred Gray had gathered a load he would throw a shore party for the divers. There would be liquor, of course, though I never took any of that. We would boil our trepang for a couple of hours, then bury it overnight in the sand away from flies and insects. Then we would boil it again for two hours. By now it would be quite soft and easy to eat. We would strip off the skin and eat it from the end like a banana. Or cut it in slices. Yolngu never got the habit of eating trepang because of all the cooking it needs. But if they knew about its sexual energy I'm sure they would be cooking it constantly. I never recommended it or encouraged it, because our people don't need to develop their sexual energy any higher than it is. Our nation is growing fast enough without that. So I kept quiet about the sexual side of trepang.

But the cut-leaf palm, or lanhu, has a growing tip that is beautiful to eat. Some people are extremely fond of it. The name Lanhupuy, as in our friend Wesley Lanhupuy, means fond of eating palm shoots. There's a smaller kind called bulmurrk. Each is beautiful to eat and

each lubricates a man's sexual strength and smoothness. Considering that the tree is lost if the shoot is eaten, this is a high price for sexual energy in a man. The Chinese esteem a little palm which they grow for its root, which they like to eat because it preserves their health and sexual energy. They call it ginseng. But that's another story.

1 Macknight, CC (1976) *The Voyage to Marege. Macassan Trepangers in Northern Australia* Melbourne University Press.

2 In December 1988, the National Congress of Indonesian Psychiatry (IDAJA) held its inaugural conference, in Ujung Pandang. I was invited to speak on a topic that completely took the wind from my sails—the 'Aggression of Aborigines'! The conference and my visit turned out to be an enthralling experience, both for me and for the three delegates from Arnhem Land whom I invited to accompany me.

3 Beaglehole, John Cawte (1966) *The Exploration of the Pacific* (third edition) Stanford University Press.

4 Flinders, M A, *Voyage to Terra Australis*. See Australiana Facsimile Editions No 37, reproduced by the Libraries Board of South Australia from an original copy held in the Public Library of South Australia Adelaide 1966.

5 Dr James Lind, 'the father of naval hygiene', at last induced the Admiralty in 1795 to issue the order that the navy be supplied with lemons. His 'A Treatise of the Scurvy' (1753) is a medical classic.

6 An exegesis of the Warramirri gods is to be found in my earlier book, Cawte J (1993) *The Universe of the Warramirri: Art, Medicine and Religion in Arnhem Land* University of New South Wales Press. This book contains coloured prints of paintings and carvings specially prepared for the text. I wrote it at their request. All royalties from sales are forwarded to them by the publisher.

the DEADLIEST jellyfish

Alec Donaldson lay on the battered co
beach. He was doing nothing, perhaps
His position resembled that of the herd
of success in Borneo had come to noth
with Donaldson it was a fishing venture
fronds of the coconut palms at the gang
in the shallows. They were creating ar
rocks and old oil drums that disfigured
had never used it.

The children in the water were doubtless cooler than he. It was a vigour-sapping humid Sunday morning in November. Nothing in the Mission moved except these children and the crows, which never perched still or kept quiet. Many of the adults had gone to the little church on the rise to sit under the ceiling fans and to rest during the service. Grown-ups never bathed in the sea for fun; they never went into it if they could help it. The Arafura is an unsafe sea, abounding in venomous marine life of many kinds.

Alec Donaldson was meditating, as usual, about the failure of his project in that little community. He had been invited to this place some 15 years before with the object of establishing a Fishing Cooperative. He was an experienced professional fisherman, and this place needed his skills. On paper it looked promising. These seas teem with fish suitable for the table. In the tidal rivers you

e lounge on the verandah of his bungalow overlooking the
oondering his own predicament in a desultory way.
f Joseph Conrad's first novel, Almayer's Folly, whose dreams
ng. With Almayer it was a trade store that had failed;
ith the Yolngu. From time to time he looked up through the
f children splashing and frolicking, immersed to their waists
normous racket playing around the disused pier made of
iis pretty beach. That jetty was yet another failure; the barges

can net the fabulous barramundi, the table fish most prized by the gourmets of Sydney and Melbourne. Chances looked bright, but everything went against him from the outset. The six plank-boats that the Mission already owned turned out to be an unserviceable fleet, their hulls rotten from shipworm, the teredo that is the scourge of anything wooden in these tepid waters. At huge expense the Mission then bought a large steel-hulled replacement craft fitted with refrigeration. Now the Yolngu did not care to work in it. They preferred the small craft, each of which could be run by a circle of brothers of the same clan. They were uneasy about going to sea with members of other clans with whom they had old grievances and scores to settle. The steel-hulled vessel now lay rusting in the mud on the leeward side of the island, not used. But that was only one of many setbacks.

The freezing and packing factory which the missionaries installed on the beach, constructed of galvanized iron sheets, had an old refrigeration plant which was hard to maintain. The refrigeration kept breaking down, and if ever their frozen product thawed, it had to be thrown out. There was no money left to install a new plant. Their basic economic disadvantage was of course the distance. They had to fly out their frozen fish by the commercial airlines, and their main markets were a thousand miles away. This made their business non-competitive with fisheries operating closer to the big markets.

Even the government seemed to obstruct them. Once there had been an outbreak of typhoid fever in the township, and the public health authority had closed down the factory and kept it closed for six devastating months. Everybody lost heart after that.

On top of all this, the Arafura Sea is a hellish place to work: some of its species are the most venomous in the world. That is why the adults never enter the water if they can help it. The beach where the children were now playing was reasonably safe, especially when the wind ruffled the surface and the water was clear. Marine stingers frequent the calm and murky water that is more likely to contain the small animals they capture by paralysing them with their stinging cells, before digesting them as food. No, the fishing industry had turned out a fiasco where high hopes once were held. All very demoralizing for a fisherman who had been invited here to develop it.

An ear-splitting scream shattered his ruminations. Some children were struggling up out of the water onto the beach as fast as they could get there. They scrambled out naked for the most part. Three of them ran back into the water to assist a child who seemed hardly able to stand, and was being left behind in the mad scramble. They let her fall on the wet sand at the edge of the lapping waves and clustered around, still screaming. Alec Donaldson stood up on his verandah craning his neck to see what was happening. Was it one of his kids?—that was his first thought. The stricken child was too dark. He saw a boy try to wipe the child's chest to clear something away, then withdraw his hand with a scream of pain. He plunged a couple of fingers into his mouth, which hurt his lips so much that he yelped like a dog and ran about in a state of frantic distraction.

By this time it was obvious to Donaldson what was happening. He rocketed down the steps of his verandah and leaped down the rugged hill to the beach, his bare feet plunging across the boulders.

The stricken child was an eight-year-old girl whom he recognized instantly. She was wearing the briefest of vees over her hips; the rest of her body and face were draped with grey cords, the detached tentacles of a box jellyfish adhering fast to her dark skin. She lay on her back without moving or uttering a sound, in contrast to the screaming children pressing around her. Her eyes were open but her face wore no expression at all; she had completely collapsed, and Donaldson wondered if she were dead.

Alec pelted back up the hill to fetch his truck and slammed it recklessly down to the beach. With a blanket he lifted the child aboard and headed for the nurse's aid post. The little girl seemed dead already to him, but he laid her on his blanket on the examination table to await the nurse, who had to be called from the church.

The first act of the nurse was to lock the door of the surgery to keep out the crowd of onlookers. She poured vinegar over the adherent tentacles and wiped away their jelly with a towel. She could detect no pulse, no heartbeat, no breathing. But when she tried the ultimate sign of death, inserting a wisp of the girl's hair into her open eye, she thought she detected a flicker, a reflex closure of the lids: perhaps some nervous activity remained after all? A throng of faces watched her every move through the window.

She positioned an oxygen mask over the little girl's face and respired her by compressing the bag. She massaged the heart. Still the child made no response. She got Alec Donaldson to carry on with the emergency procedures he had watched her doing while she flew to the radio to summon the Health Department plane from the town, 200 miles away across the uninhabited bays and islands. As luck would have it there was a plane waiting on the ground, and it took off right away. The child was shortly evacuated to the town hospital, but she was indeed dead on the trip, as the nurse knew in her heart. But to send her off seemed the wisest course; it gave some hope, and some time for the crisis to settle.

The *Sydney Morning Herald* somehow learned of it; the paper featured a small paragraph about a child being killed by the deadly 'sea wasp' while bathing in shallow water at this Mission township. Not an important item, or an unusual occurrence, as several deaths occur every year; but these news items serve to remind readers that it is unsafe to swim in the tropical waters in summer. If you must enter the water, keep your clothes on and your skin covered.

I learned the identity of the dead child when I arrived for my annual visit as a volunteer doctor a few weeks later. She was my own grandchild, in terms of the family ties that had been bestowed on me years before: a Warramirri girl of the northern islands, the daughter of the eldest son of my brother and closest friend. Soon I learned of the web of maledictions and recriminations that now enmeshed this tragedy.

Death from the stings of sea wasps is not seen as an accident or a misadventure. Only the very young or old die naturally; everybody else is killed. Who had instigated this death? Who sent the sea wasp to sting that child? That was the question everybody was asking. An autopsy had been conducted at the town hospital 200 miles away, with the sanction of closest family members. It disclosed nothing that they did not know. That was how the event came to the notice of the reporter and the *Herald*. A Morning Star ceremony was conducted as soon as the girl's body came back for the burial, to help speed the ghost to *Bralgu*, the Isle of the Dead. The ghost may have been dispelled but suspicion proliferated.

Some of the blame being handed out was directed at the nurse. She was being accused, on the report of those who had watched her through the window hard at work trying to revive the child, for wiping the jellyfish off the skin with a towel. This would only have forced more tentacles into closer contact with the skin, discharging more venom. She should have scraped the jelly off lightly with a knife! On the other hand she was applauded for pouring on vinegar and not alcohol as most of the poisoning manuals then advised. Those who have been stung are confident that vinegar is more effective in destroying the venom and in reducing the pain. Alec Donaldson thought that the box jellyfish had come in close to the sheltered water in the lee of that damned pier. Before the pier was made, this open beach had a safe record for not attracting sea wasps. He blamed the lack of funds which had prevented them constructing a proper pier with pillars instead of having to dump rocks and masonry to make a breakwater. But these complaints were mere matters of fact and so, unimportant.

The real question at stake was not so much who was the fiend who wanted this poor child to die in the fullness of her carefree days. Rather the question was: who was the enemy of the family who wanted its mother to weep, to mourn, to gash her temples and scalp until they bled freely in her public lamentation, as was required of her?

Beyond all that, who was the enemy who wanted the husband-to-be in the Galpu clan, awaiting this girl for whom he had made bride payments all these years, to be flung into frustration and anger at being so cruelly robbed? Who should take the blame for this, and bear the brunt of Galpu pay-back?

In discussions of these questions an answer presented itself that seemed to resolve these matters to the satisfaction of most of the protagonists. Not long after the child's burial, her father arrived in his boat from an outer island, together with the white woman with whom he consorted. He had got there as soon as the news reached him. Blame was now directed at that white woman. She had stolen this man a couple of years before from his true wife, the mother of his children, including this child now dead. They had fled the island and they lived as exiles. She was leading him on a life of adventure in their boat, up and down this coastline, some of the time in the deserted islands of his ancestors.

Such a life called for plenty of courage and resourcefulness on her part, it seemed to me. She was a remarkable woman, this white woman, who had been inspired to elope with this man out of a sense of excitement and tropical island romance, of the kind that made The Swiss Family Robinson the popular reading matter of her childhood. Western life had become deadeningly humdrum for her: she had turned her back on it, for this.

The arrival of this pair of romantics back on the island provided the gossips with a convenient solution. When they stepped ashore the white woman was roundly assailed and reviled for contributing to the child's death by abducting its father. She was not per-mitted to stay ashore; she was forced to return to live on the boat at anchor in the stream. In a few days they departed. When they returned a second time after the lapse of a few months she was permitted ashore and the matter was allowed to rest, though her welcome was always cool in many quarters. This woman bore all this opprobrium like a stoic; one had to admire her for it.

But there was a deeper, darker story going the rounds that the child's death was nothing to do with this white woman. On one level, this story blamed the new coterie of Christian missionaries for enticing the mothers of the township to attend church on that Sunday morning, leading them to neglect to supervise their children who had thereby been left open to this sea wasp attack. How sinister that it had occurred during divine service! Clearly the missionaries had not done this with malice aforethought; they were too transparent in their good intentions. No, they were being used; it was a *raggalk*, a sorcerer, who had sung to the preacher to hold the service and had compelled the women to attend the church and leave their children exposed to risk. Every weather forecast on the radio at that time uttered a warning that sea wasps were close in shore, everywhere in the Territory. They all neglected to listen to the warning or to heed it.

Levels beneath levels! On an even more hidden level, this death was being linked with two previous deaths in the Galpu clan. Folk had died from attacks by shark and crocodile, and now by this sea wasp. Who was signalling these savage creatures to attack? Gossip pointed to one hostile clan which shall be nameless. Gossip suggested that when a fourth calamity should occur, there was going to be wholesale pay-back for all that filthy magic. The older men were credited with understanding the source of life and death. When those enemy Yolngu want to do something evil they sing to the blood of people who have died, which they bring out from its hiding place. Then that dead person's spirit, the *morkoi*, commands *gaywarr*, the sea wasp, to close in for the kill.

I could not avoid hearing maledictions and imprecations. Here is one that I copied down.

Song: Sea Wasp, Attack!

Ngayam djangu gaywarr
I am that sea wasp
Ngayam djangu raitjung
I am that jelly fish
Marwarr lawurrba
The power of the sea, essence of the sea
Guntjirryirr wilingarr
Poisonous jellyfish, agonizing jellyfish!
Nhadini gululangurr buwanatji ngurru
I can calm waves of the shallows, and the
deep ocean
Gundhuma
Out where the clouds rise in April
Galiyan wurrugu
I am the furnace, the oven of the ocean

When the *raggalk* sings this song, smoke rises from the blood of the dead, they say, and forms the spirit which takes the evil instruction to this poisonous assailant, launching him on his attack.

'Out where the clouds rise in April I am the furnace, the oven of the ocean.' How is it possible for such a malevolent song, a song of cursing and terror, to be couched in such poetry? Perhaps, you may say, all poetry that has such power must have a breath of sorcery in it. Unlikely! Poetry does not turn people against each other in a

tumult of suspicion and rumor; it enlightens and purifies. How I wished that I could enlighten these people about the pure chance of the sea wasp! It may be one of the most sinister denizens of the sea, yet it has its place in nature and a poetry of its own. Let me describe its characteristics from a medical point of view and ask the reader to judge—which is more miraculous, its demonology or its zoology?

It is correct to call the sea wasp a kind of nettle. The phylum Cnidaria, distinguished by its cnidoblast or stinging cell, takes its name from the Greek for knife, or nettle. The stinging cell holds ready the nematocyst (Greek: *nematos*, a thread) as its offensive weapon. Most coelenterates—jellyfish, corals, sea-anemones, hydras—have a nematocyst of varying degrees

The box jellyfish or sea wasp has four bundles of long stinging tentacles.

of power. Nature has given them these stinging cells to paralyse small animals that swim within their reach. This is the way they capture and digest their food. Unfortunately nature has not given them the means to discriminate these small animals from the skin of humans. They are like venomous snakes, wasting their venom on an object too large to swallow as food.

The nematocyst is a tiny grenade, an explosive device with a very sensitive fuse pin. In its resting position the stinging cell is a sac of venom smaller than the head of a pin, with its projectile parts coiled up inside. These parts include a barb or spicule which can pierce the skin when it ejects from the cell. Then the long hollow thread that is coiled around it is unleashed to wander in the wound, discharging a venom like a miniature hypodermic syringe.

The Chironex jelly-fish with which we are concerned has tentacles that drift behind its body for as much as several metres. All of them are lined with nematocysts ready to discharge. A remarkable range, when you realise that the main body measures ten centimetres across! This body is shaped like a bell, hence the name cubo-medusa or box jellyfish. Medusa conveys its character better than jellyfish, if it recalls the Gorgon slain by Perseus who wisely looked at its reflection, not its face.

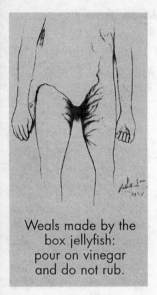

Weals made by the box jellyfish: pour on vinegar and do not rub.

The nematocyst is triggered to explode when a fine sentinel hair on the exposed side brushes against a living prey. If the prey is a vertebrate—like a small girl—the venom floods the wounds and enters the bloodstream, promptly reaching the nervous system. Like snake venom it is neurotoxic before all else. The envenomation depends on the extent of the wound and the quantity of venom. It depends on the season; late in summer the jelly-fish is sexually mature and more active. And it depends on the nutritional state of victim and attacker alike. A massive attack brings on muscular paralysis and respiratory failure, as in our small girl. Death can occur in under a minute. For those who recover, the weals remain extremely painful.

Chironex fleckeri is the most dan-gerous jellyfish in any sea of the world. For this it is called the deadly sea wasp. It abounds close inshore in turbid water after the monsoonal rains bring their food-bearing run-off. Being hyaline in appearance it is virtually invisible in such water, although it leaves a shadow on the sandy bed below. Its wounds on exposed skin are long weals that look as if they could have been made by repeated lashes with a stockwhip.

As a first aid measure, the blubber should be scraped off with a knife, not wiped off, which only triggers more nematocysts to fire. The best lotion is vinegar, which seems to neutralize the venom better than the alcohol which the medical books used to recommend. Antivenene should be stocked in all first aid cabinets in these zones and should be injected immediately, even before the artificial respiration and cardiac massage are set in train. When the victim responds, cortisone may reduce the pain and swelling of the weals. Since young children along these coasts will inevitably get into the sea in summer, whatever the warnings, immunizing them with a toxoid serum available from the Commonwealth Serum Laboratories is not a bad idea. This is also recommended for adults whose jobs involve immersing themselves in these dangerous waters.

By comparison with the lethal Chironex, the other marine stingers are merely unpleasant at best and painful at worst. *Physalia physalis*, the Portuguese man-o-war or bluebottle, is encountered worldwide. You will often find them on the beach, blown ashore by the wind; they are named for the inflated 'sail' that rides on the surface, trailing their dark-blue tentacles below. Cyanea, commonly called snotty or brown blubber, is also a denizen of the world's seas, common in the Atlantic, moderately painful but less dangerous. The mauve stinger called *Pelagia noctiluca* is more prevalent in subtropical waters; its name *noctiluca* is derived from its phosphorescence.

If you have cause to be concerned about the danger of the tropic shallows you can find all this and much more in many books. But if you want to learn what the people who are at risk make of it you must go to them, as we have just gone to the people of the Arafura Sea. If they ask for your advice, it will do no good to dilate on the medical zoology, as the books do and I have done. But there is one good piece of advice to offer. Considering how vicious the venom is, it is a matter for wonder that the deadly sea wasp could have any natural enemies. But it does. That extraordinary and harmless animal the turtle is able to eat it without any discomfort. Turtles must have the toughest gullet in the animal kingdom. But the number of turtles is being depleted by hunting and more especially by raids on their egg nests in

the sandhills beside the beach. If turtles must be hunted, never rob their nests. The turtle population is our best protection. It feeds on jellyfish. The fewer turtles, the more stingers, leading to more dead children, and more feuding over their deaths by people constantly reckoning with curses and pay-back.

Alec Donaldson was a competent professional fisherman, with enough grasp of marine biology to know that the turtle is the natural enemy of the stinger. But he could never come to grips with Yolngu magical thinking, the very personality characteristic that had undermined the success of his Fishing Cooperative. It baffled his powers of comprehension that the same people who would impute a little girl's death to malice rather than to misadventure were a people who would tolerate the mishaps of an infant Fishing Cooperative, not blaming a soul for incompetence. Joseph Conrad's hero is not an isolated instance of a defeated man in these waters, where there must be a legion of Almayers, and their Follies.

There is a chihuahua plant i
against it you are taken to ho
America. Early Portuguese na
ous fish poisoning they met i
range across the coral seas of th

VIRULEN

While visiting Elcho Island in June 1977 I heard that the big man Wattle Tree, the leader of the Galpu clan, had recently been rushed to Gove Hospital suffering from ciguatera fish poisoning—along with fourteen other men, all on the same afternoon. It must have been quite an afternoon for the admitting medical officer at that little hospital. Happily he did not have to contend with preliminary paperwork like health insurance. It appeared that Wattle Tree had not partaken too heavily of the poisoned fish, because he was able to recover quickly, escape from hospital and return home to Elcho Island. Later I sat with him, under the big mango tree that shaded his cottage on the Galpu side of the Mission township, to learn his story about this fish poisoning. He ceremonially caused a new blanket to be produced for me to sit on. He did not want

exico reputed to be so deadly that if you so much as brush
tal. It is the ciguatera, the scourge of the plains of South
tors adopted its name, ciguatera, for an equally danger-
pic waters. This sea scourge now seems to be extending its
cific where it is causing much concern.

fish

the doctor sitting on the ground!

I never knew a Yolngu patriarch with so many wives, or better room service, than the august Wattle Tree.

He picked up from his rug his Macassan pipe, a hollow tube a full yard long, bearing a machine-gun cartridge shell at the end. This served for the burner, into which he stuffed the Three Nuns I had brought him as a present. He could inhale the smoke of the entire barrel in a single breath, without losing consciousness, though of course he only did this while recumbent. After he recovered from the asphyxia, he proceeded to tell me the story of the fish poisoning. He was happy to see me, because although he had recovered from the more severe

effects in the hospital, he was still far from feeling well. His muscles ached. His hands and feet itched and tingled. He looked slow and depressed. And it was now a month since he was poisoned by eating that fish. He asked if I might have some medicine for this misery? It so happened that I did. We were all happy that it helped him. We shall come to my remedy later.

Wattle Tree had been taking a vacation from his domestic duties at Yirrkala, another Aboriginal township east of these thirty-four islands—not in the Arafura Sea at all, but rather within the Gulf of Carpentaria. Yirrkala nestles by a creek flowing into the northern waters of the Gulf. When the missionary Wilbur Chaseling[1] founded this Mission in 1936 he did not know that not far inland there was a huge deposit of bauxite, a source of that valuable ore alumina, from which aluminium is refined. He makes no mention of any such awareness in *Yulengor*, his book describing the foundation of the Mission at Yirrkala. It was known that bauxite was present in vast quantities in the Wessel Islands, but the forbidding terrain made it unlikely that it would ever be mined and exported. Open cut mining of bauxite began after the war in the Pacific, in 1962, placing great strains upon Yirrkala Mission, giving rise to the mining company town of Nhulunbuy with its smelting works and the base hospital in which Wattle Tree had just been treated. The advent of mining to this region split political opinion down the middle, in both the Yolngu and the missionary camps. Some thought the mining could provide valuable work, training and experience, but others thought these things were premature and would be the bane of their life. The latter point of view is strongly expressed in a book by another missionary, Edgar Wells.[2]

Wattle Tree enjoyed his holiday at Yirrkala until some of his kinsmen caught three big kingfish—from an aluminium dinghy, as fate ironically ordained—in Yirrkala Bay just off the little Mission township. They gutted the big fish, cut them into sections and cooked them by boiling in four-gallon oil drums over their open fire. Wattle Tree told me that everybody ate them for supper at sundown, but clearly this could not be literally true since only men were affected. The women and children were spared; they were not included in that dinner party. That night, Wattle Tree felt pains and

cramps in his stomach and when he got up to try to ease the pain he felt nauseated and he vomited. He did not sleep because in addition to the cramps in his belly his entire body ached, every single muscle of it.

Next morning he did not vomit but he was most unwell. He found it hard even to get his breath. His arms and legs were weak and he could hardly stand erect. He felt a numbness in his hands, feet and mouth, especially in his mouth. His head felt strange, as if nothing were real. All around him the other men who had shared the catch were in similar states of alarm and distress. They sent for the Mission nurse to come to help them. She took one look at them and phoned the doctor at the hospital. He exclaimed, 'Ciguatera! I'll send the ambulance!' They were able to cram the fifteen sickest men into the ambulance, which rushed them to the hospital where they were all admitted.

Wattle Tree told me that the doctor ordered injections for him. I do not know what the drug was; it may have been nikethamide to assist his breathing. After two nights in the hospital he was well enough to escape. He was the first one to escape, he told me proudly. Yolngu are rarely discharged from hospital—they escape, because in their view a hospital is a place in which to die. Escape as soon as you can! The other men were there a little longer before they were able to run away. Wattle Tree did recall that the doctor had spoken to him, telling him that he would be all right, but that he should not take any more liquor after this poisoning.

At home now, Wattle Tree was listless and inert, never leaving his rug. This was unlike him; the previous year when I visited him he escorted me into the bush to show me how the old men practised harming as well as healing, and he permitted the friend who sometimes accompanied me, camera-man Douglass Baglin, to film them in their magic circle. These are movie sequences that I sometimes show privately. I would never show them publicly lest believers in sorcery see them and conduct the deadly manoeuvres.

Now Wattle Tree sat on the rug, complaining of aching muscles, itching skin and tingling of his fingers and toes. Observing his miserable state, I prescribed the suggested medication, amitriptyline. The response was marvellous! If I believed in miracles I could have called it miraculous. Wattle Tree's unpleasant sensations were nearly gone by morning, and did not trouble him thereafter. It happened too quickly to be attributed to the central anti-depressant effect of this drug. It more resembled its immediate effect on the complaint of bedwetting. I doubt if it was a placebo response; anybody less like a placebo-reactor than Wattle Tree I have yet to meet. I have since used amitriptyline for one other victim of residual or protracted symptoms of ciguatera poisoning. I understand that there are doctors in North Queensland who are also impressed with this usage. This little piece of clinical information is not to be found in the textbooks of medicine, but it is worth knowing if you fish in the tropics or even if you eat fish from the coral reefs.

From the medical and economic standpoint, ciguatera is the most dominant type of fish poisoning in the world. The poisonous fish cannot be recognized, for they look perfectly healthy. About 300 species of fish have now been incriminated, mostly the larger ones weighing three kilograms or more.

In Australian tropical waters they include mackerel, snapper, coral trout, coral cod, sea perch, sea bass, sweetlip, red emperor and barracuda. I understand that turtles can also be affected, which is of more interest to Yolngu than to whites, who are prohibited from catching turtles. I do not know about crocodiles, but I do not see why they should be exempt. The condition is harmless to the fish themselves, only dangerous to people who eat them. We have seen that it is not a new disease, notwithstanding its recent spread, having been given its Portuguese name, ciguatera, by Ferdinand Magellan.[3] He encountered it in the Philippines and deemed it so deadly that he conferred upon it the name of that South American weed as the strongest warning he could think of.

Talking with Wattle Tree and recalling all that cursing he had taught me, I might have expected that he would blame ciguatera poisoning upon borrpoi or nyirra, that sinister bag of tricks that jealous people direct at each other in secret, hoping to summon sickness. Not a bit of it! Wattle Tree and every other Yolngu were clear that this disease arrived in their region only after the mining company's chemical works started up, and is only found in its vicinity. It was not known before that. They had to find a name for it, gunampi, because they had not heard of the Portuguese or accepted medical name for it, ciguatera.

Yolngu consider that gunampi is a sickness from coral fish, guya garrung, who are living on dead coral, rakung garrung. They believe that poison from the chemical plant runs into the sea and kills the coral on the nearest island, Bremer Island, and its reefs. Sometimes it runs on in the tide as far north as Cape Wilberforce or as far south as Yirrkala Bay. They drew a map of their *gunampi* waters, where the coral is dying, ciguatera is endemic, and you never know whether or not a fish you catch will poison you.

The toxin itself is produced by algae, such as the dinoflagellate *Gambierdiscus toxicus*, which blooms on dead coral. These algae are eaten by the small herbivorous fish, which are the prey of the larger carnivorous fish

like the mackerel. The poison ciguatoxin which these larger fish concentrate, is more potent than cyanide, weight for weight. It distresses the gut of the fish eater within a few hours of eating, then it affects the nervous system, causing a range of reactions from acute delirium to delayed nerve palsy. This latter causes the bizarre sensations of which the victims often complain.

In the longer run, it may cause an

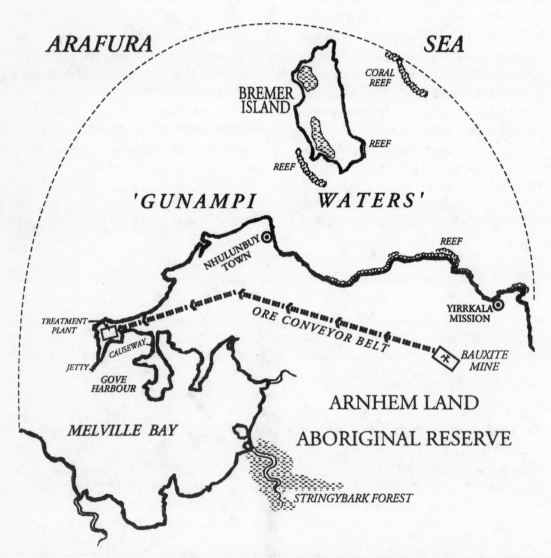

CIGUATERA (GUNAMPI) POISONING WATERS

BY MOYNYU, BURRUMARRA, WANDJUK MARIKA

asthenic condition with insomnia, irritability, fatigue and depression. This syndrome can endure for months, and exacerbations can be triggered by eating fish—even good fish—or by taking alcohol. Wattle Tree's hospital doctor had given him sound advice. These victims are sometimes diagnosed as neurotic. But they may in fact be undergoing a serious complication of ciguatoxin: a delayed allergic demyelination, in which the lining of peripheral nerves dies back.

Coral is like a beautiful woman: people gaze at it, idealize it and romanticize its beauty. A physician-poet, Richard Garnett, is typical of people living in cold climes who romanticize the coral reefs of the *zonae torridae*.

> The deeps have music soft and low
> When winds awake the airy spry.
> It lures me, lures me on to go
> And see the land where corals lie,
> The land where corals lie …

The poem by Dr Garnett, set to music by Sir Edward Elgar, says something about the fascination of coral. Hear it sung by Dame Janet Baker, contralto, and you can almost picture coral in its living form, so different from the skeletons in museums and old-fashioned drawing rooms. But hear a Yolngu sing Nulwardo's song:

> *Ngayam djangu ngulwado,*
> *djinaku manguyngawu*
> I am this coral being, this ocean being

> *Djinal ngayangarru manbuyngawu*
> *nguya*
> Here I shall be the ocean being
> living in

> *Wabululwu, ratjkuka rratjnga; ngayam*
> *ngulwado.*

> The breakers, reef spray and the tides; I
> am the coral being.

> *Ngayam maday, ngayam manda,*
> *ngayam manbuynga.*
> I am the crayfish, I am the octopus, I am
> the ocean being.

> *Ngayam rranggurra, ngayam djabana,*
> *ngayam dirrmalla.*

> I am the calm water, I am the red cloud,
> I am the north wind.

Yolngu think coral generates species, up as far as humanity. Our Warramirri are a clan of sailors, who paddled between thirty-four islands, and sometimes sailed. I have found that they have a theory of evolution resembling that of Darwin, in which life began in the form of the lowly coral animals, which underwent a series of changes into higher forms, at length to human form. These changes were supervised by the sea god Marryalyan. An amusing god, always busy changing shapes and colours: Marryalyan the metamorphoser.

I found this theory of evolution surprising because it is different from that held by inland or freshwater indigenes, whose gods created the natural forms at one marvellous stroke, like the god of Abraham and Moses. I no longer find it disconcerting because in the meantime I have grown a little more familiar with the Arafura Sea and the thirty-four islands. Between the tides, on the reefs, under the waves, life here is constant change. There would have to be a change theory to account for it.

Look at corals more closely. No species alters its appearance more, before one's very eyes, than the coelenterates. The Arafura Sea is the sea of the phylum Coelenterata, the corals and anemones. These animals are everywhere to be seen, and so are their cousins, the jellyfish. The coelenterates are simple animals, basically just a maw, lined by two layers of cells, ectoderm outside and endoderm inside. Around the mouth are tentacles that have contractile cells, with presumably some form of nervous conduction, enabling the tentacles to extend, entrap the prey and draw it into the cavity of the body. The corals and anemones are mostly fixed to the reef, the jellyfish floating above.

No garden ever devised by human hand can match the colours of the reef garden, the rainbow trail beneath the sea. All the hues of the rainbow are mixed in dazzling profusion most wonderfully, in a living, muscular, sinuous movement. No garden is so dangerous, with flowers fitted with needles which sting, paralyse and kill their prey. The nematocysts of the coelenterates of these waters are triggered to fire their weapon at the slightest touch. The sea wasp is deadly to humans. Marryalyan's living coral is colourful, writhing, changing, growing before your eyes. To these reef-dwellers it is Nulwardo,[4] the origin of life. Dead coral specimen is merely calcium carbonate, like dead bone. But dead, it is more dangerous. Its skeleton provides the base for planktonic algae to proliferate.

It does not surprise me that the people of these islands should hold a theory of evolution roughly resembling the one which Charles Darwin developed, sailing the coast of South America and the Galapagos in HMS Beagle. We now know that there are weaknesses in Darwin's theory. At that time there was no knowledge of inheritance through genes (genetics), nor of mutations occurring in the

genes, some of which might endow the animal with favourable characteristics for survival. Nor can we say that Darwin was first to think of evolution. He recorded more observations to fit the theory.

However, if we listen to the inhabitants of the Arafura Sea, they ask us to consider gunampi (ciguatera) as Nulwardo's sickness, a visitation from the white man. Here and there in the Pacific Ocean and its many seas, patches of coral are dying. The fish which live around dead coral, though they do not seem to be sick themselves, may poison the people who catch them for food. It is ciguatera poisoning. Fortunately, there is none of it in the vicinity of the Warramirri's islands, but as we have seen there is plenty of it a little further east, from Cape Wilberforce south to the white town of Nhulunbuy and the black Yirrkala settlement.

Wattle Tree drew me a map of how they see their gunampi waters. Coral! The coral being, Nulwardo, is tender, very easily injured, and if he declines, so does his fisherman and—who knows?—the calm water, the red cloud and the north wind, those other images of Nulwardo.

After I treated Wattle Tree, I checked the medical literature to see where the scientists were with ciguatera research. Dr Takeshi Yasumoto, a consultant of the World Health Organization, announced in Manila in 1977 that destruction of coral reefs, such as by dredging or building piers, is triggering the outbreaks of ciguatera poisoning. According to Dr Yasumoto, minute algae which live in coral reefs are provoked to multiply when the environment is disturbed. It spreads over the dead coral. Little fish feed on

Marngitj (medicine man) in the Arafura Swamps

We have landed at a small airstrip at an outstation called Arafura Swamp, among the billabongs of the Goyder River which runs northward towards Milingimbi Island. I came here in a Cessna piloted by Rev. Harold Shepherdson ('Sheppie'), the 'flying missionary'. The purpose of my visit is to see a child who may be suffering from yaws, and if necessary to return the child with its mother for treatment at the Mission. Sheppie encourages Yolngu people to stay at their remote outstations, rather than to move camp to the large settlement where tobacco is always obtainable. He knows that tobacco is highly addictive, and that most users, once hooked, will leave home to get it. So he flies tobacco to them in his Cessna. Without this, they would undoubtedly move to town where there is nothing for them to do! At the Mission's church, Rev. Shepherdson has just played to this little band a tape recording of a church service, conducted in Yolngu.

I talk to Djipuru, the marrigitj (medicine man) of this little clan. His English is very limited, but we have the help of another man who tries to interpret the comments as we discuss the child's illness. Djipuru's theatrical gestures are of the highest significance here. He is blaming the attack of the yaws on spite and malice of the neighbours in the paperbark forest which lies on the horizon. His small clan has been sung, or cursed, from some raggalk (sorcerer) who bears a grudge against Djipuru's clan. Djipuru says that the villain should be deterred and paid back. Most of their illnesses result from malice of this kind.

Djipuru has extracted his hidden amulet from the woven string bag so that it lies in front of him. This is the pay-back implement that he commands—a small wooden carving with two projecting horns of the water buffalo.

A beast rife in these wet lands, the water buffalo (*Bubalis bubalis*) was introduced from Indonesia over 100 years ago. As a domestic beast of burden, it was intended for use as a drudge at the Northern Territory settlements, for ploughing and carrying tasks like, the curabao in the Philippines and South-East Asia. These settlements survived only a few years, however. Heat, disease and crop failures had their effects and the colonies were abandoned, leaving the terrain to the imported herds of cattle, pigs and water buffalo.

The monsoonal lowlands of Northern Territory offered these invaders a readymade niche in which they thrived. Their wallowing turned wetlands into muddy bogs, and their systematic rampage created new water channels that permitted salt to spread from the coast into the freshwater flood plains. Today, the buffalo population numbers several hundred thousand—the pigs are beyond count.

The Yolngu clan has adopted the long strong horns of this powerful animal as its weapon of retaliation against enemies who curse illness on them

Over the years, a number of Aboriginal medicine men, responding to my inquiries, have donated their medicine bags for my museum of Aboriginal medicine at Prince Henry Hospital in Sydney. Djipuru is one of these donors. The role of the marngitj is seen as vital to the clan's health, even its survival, and their bags contain secret amulets, designed to defend the clan against evil, disease and misfortune. The hospital collection includes other necromantic objects such as pointing bones, kidney fat blades and kurdaitcha (featherfoot) shoes, all having power to inflict harm, even death.

In the belief that my necromantic museum collection should be more widely available for study, I offered to donate it to a major museum in one of Australia's state capitals. It was regretfully declined. To many people, the objects in my collection represent 'the black art', and are invariably kept hidden. This might be where they should remain! For the present, the hospital will keep them.

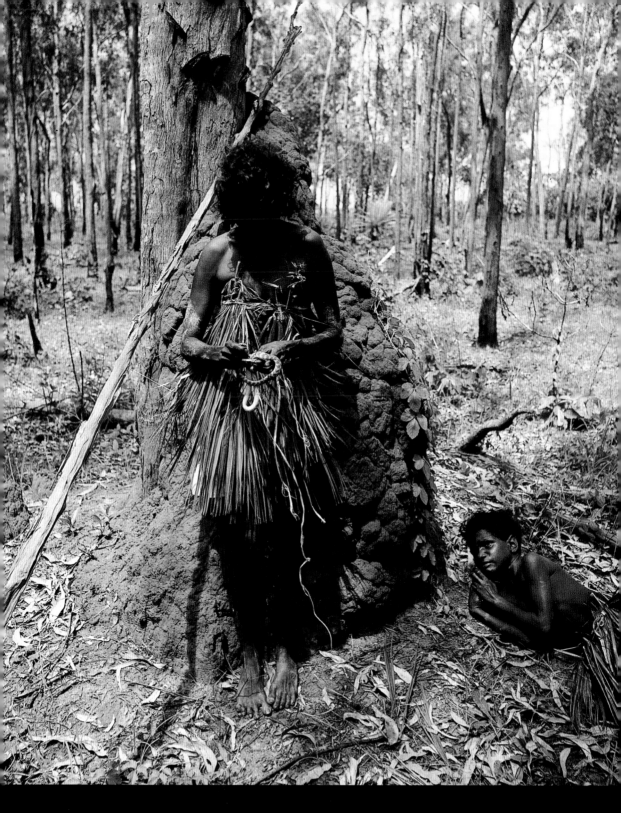

Don't run away after a snakebite!
The snake was pursued and captured with a forked stick.
It is tied, unharmed, to a tree beneath which the bitten child is made to rest.
The snake is promised release as soon as the child recovers.
Otherwise it will be killed.
A powerful bargain, inducing complete rest—in child and snake!

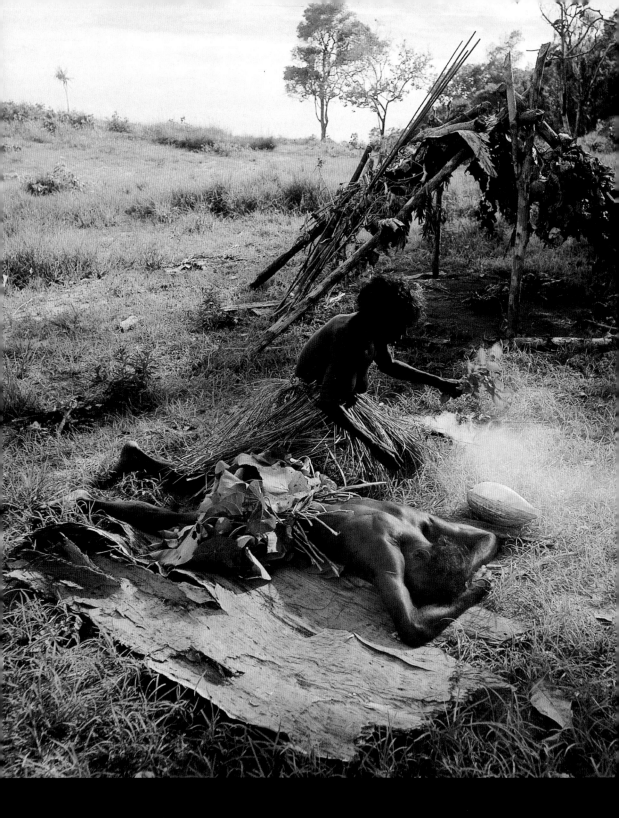

Sucking out the chest.
At a lonely camp near a beach, an older woman prepares to treat a young man
with chronic coughing.
He lies on a blanket of paperbark, beside a giant bailer shell filled with water.
A fire is lit.
Soon she will suck copious phlegm from the wall of his chest, to spit into her fire.

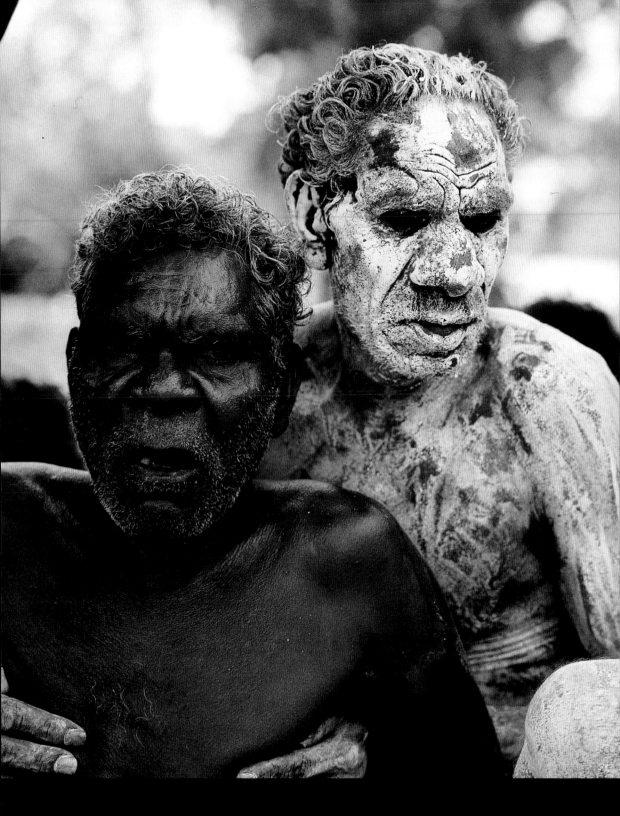

Support for the aged.
The elderly hope to elicit support and respect, even if not engaged directly in ceremonial.
This old man has been outside the ceremony; he lacks the smeared white clay of performers.
He has collapsed from emotion.
He is being tenderly raised
by a performer.

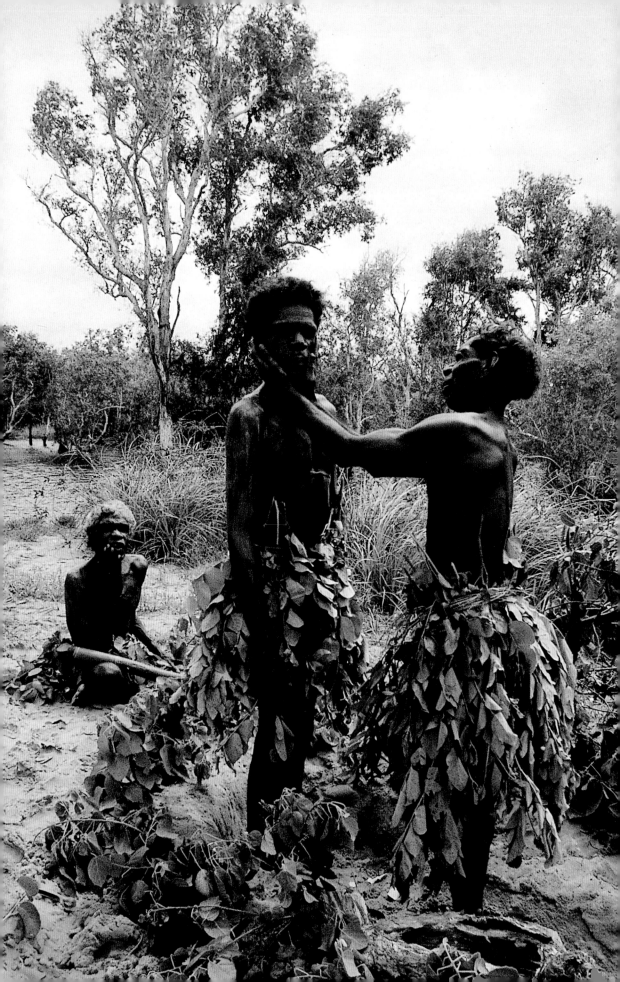

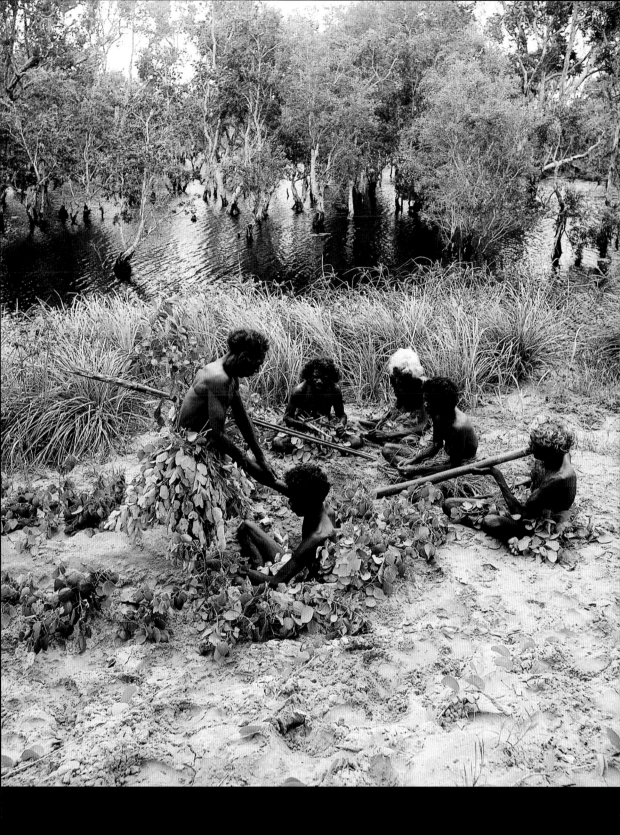

The Healing Well, Bilimbirr.
Great care has been taken to excavate by hand a sacred well in a sand dune by a billabong.
The supplicant is a man who has lost his vitality.
The marngitj ministers to him, while the chorus sings to the spirits of the earth to dispel
bad spirits. The sick man is raised from the healing well.

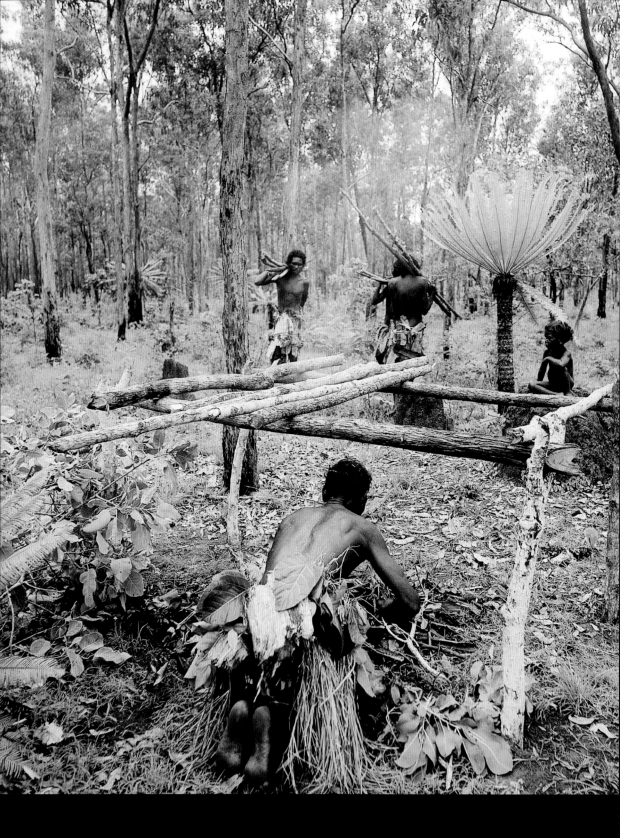

Building the Steaming Bed.
This steam bed is a raised framework, erected here in scrubland among termite castles.
The coughing man lies on top so that steam perfuses him from wet leaves
placed on the fire beneath.
The purpose is to expel the cough from the chest.

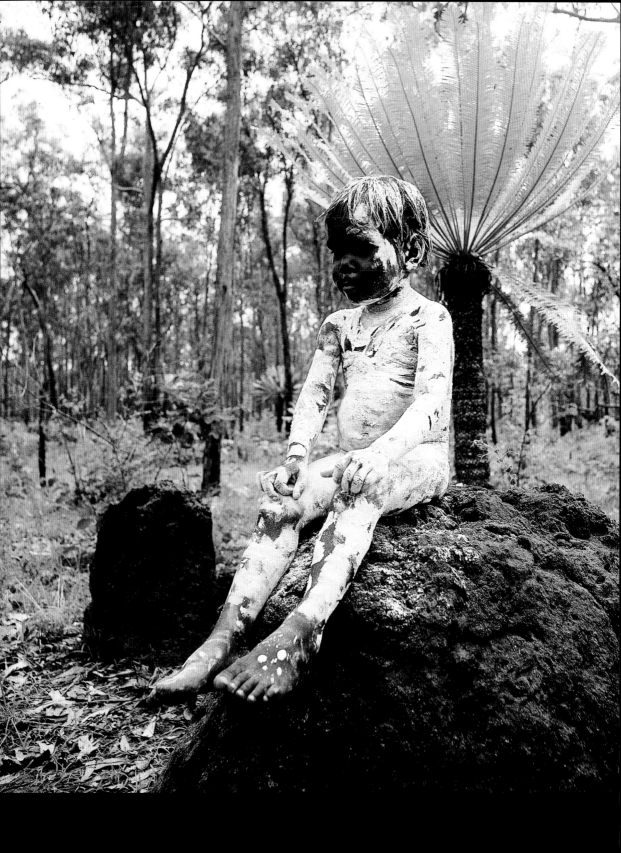

A child in training for healing.
A future medicine man is likely to be appointed while a child.
Here, a boy sits alone on an anthill, skin completely covered with white clay,
observing the procedures, hearing the songs, absorbing the mystique.

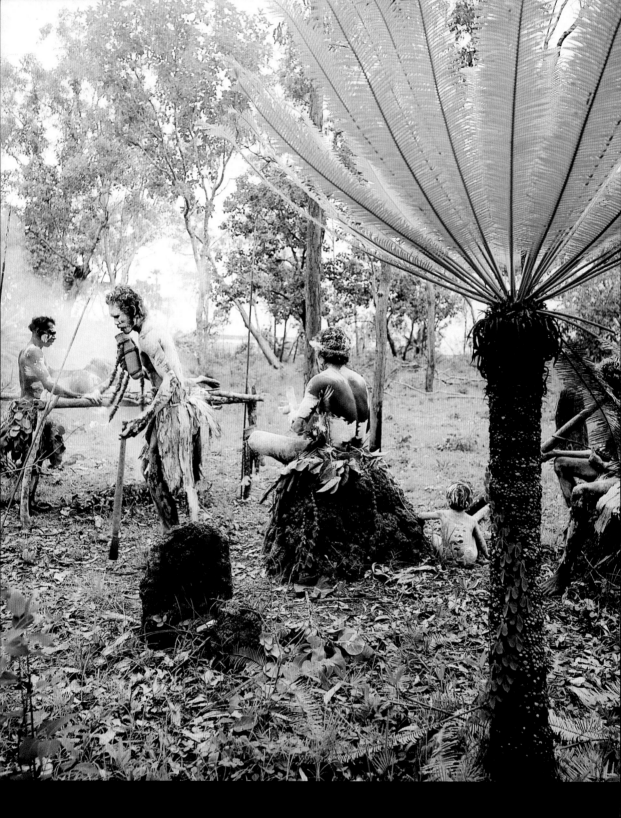

A much needed drink!
The marngitj tries to revive the subject of the steam bed with a long drink of water
from a vessel made of paperbark.
The steam bed delivers stresses to spirits in the chest.
It can be tough to ensure as a treatment.

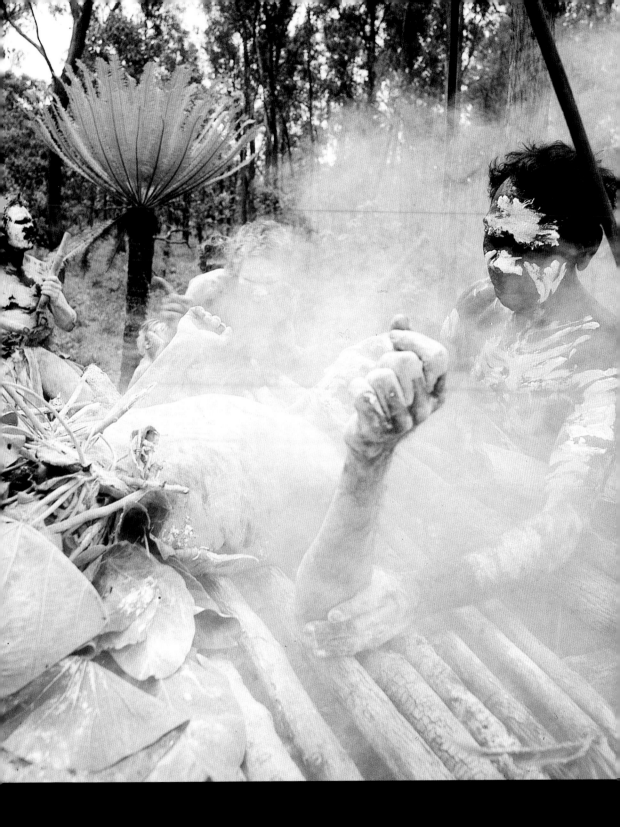

A cloud from the steam bed.
The sick man and the medicine man are immersed together in the cloud of steam—
or is it of smoke?
In fact, asphyxia was considerable; the illness worsened.
My injections were demanded to treat the deterioration the same night.

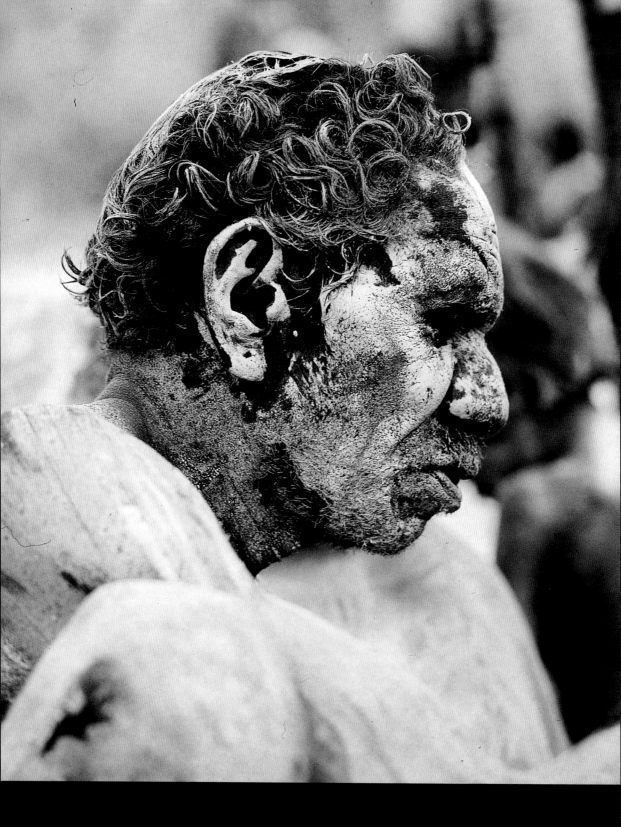

A painted face.
Kaolin clay prepares the participants in important ceremonies such as funerals.
This absorbed expression is shown as a reminder that there is no prevailing
personality type in the Yolngu: introverts are found along with extroverts.

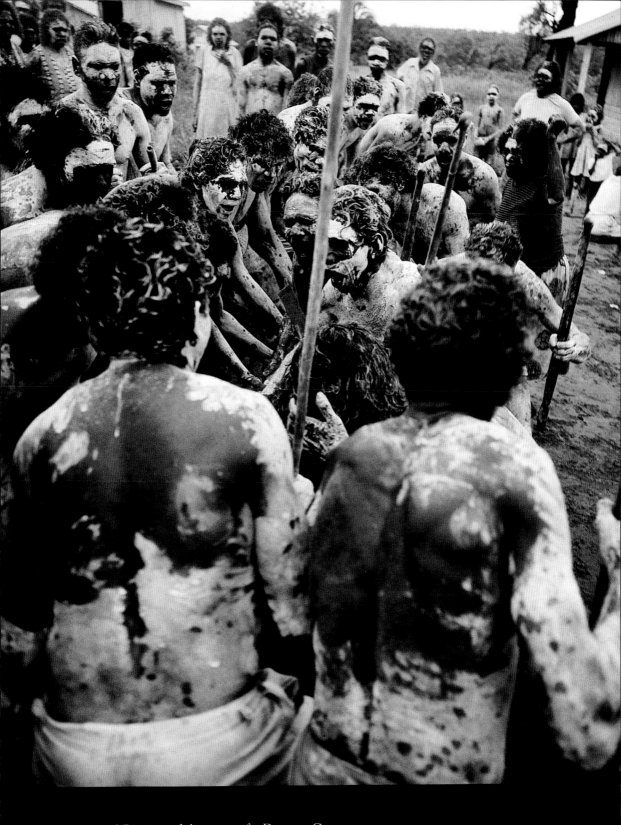

A ceremonial Raising of the mast of a Dugout Canoe.
Objects transferred from the Macassan sailors to Arnhem Land over recent centuries are classified as belonging to the Yirritja moiety.
They include seagoing canoes and their masts.
Raising the mast at a funeral symbolises the spirit's departure to the northern lands of the dead.

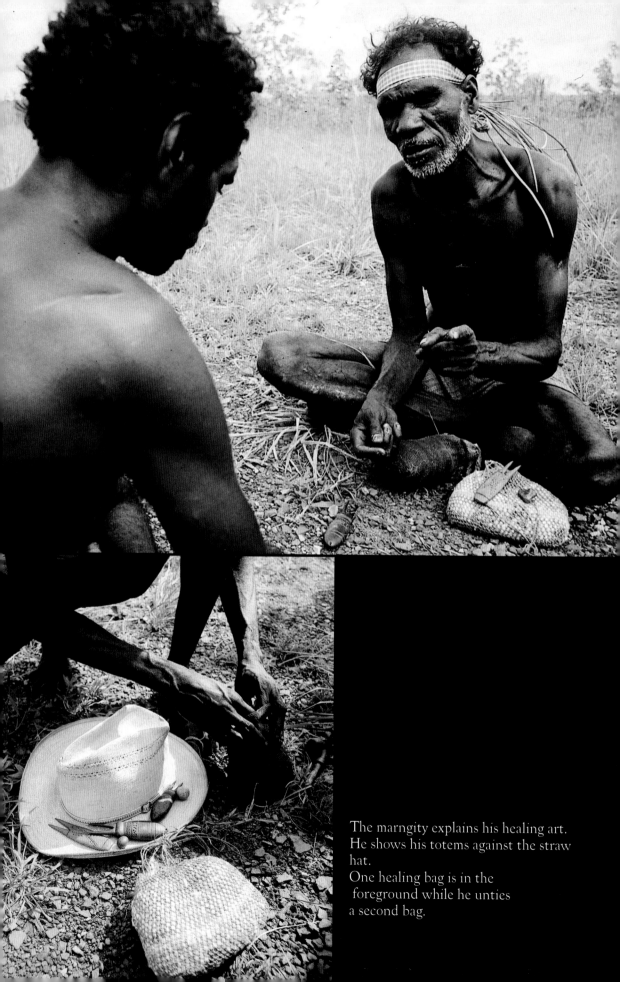

The marngity explains his healing art.
He shows his totems against the straw
hat.
One healing bag is in the
 foreground while he unties
a second bag.

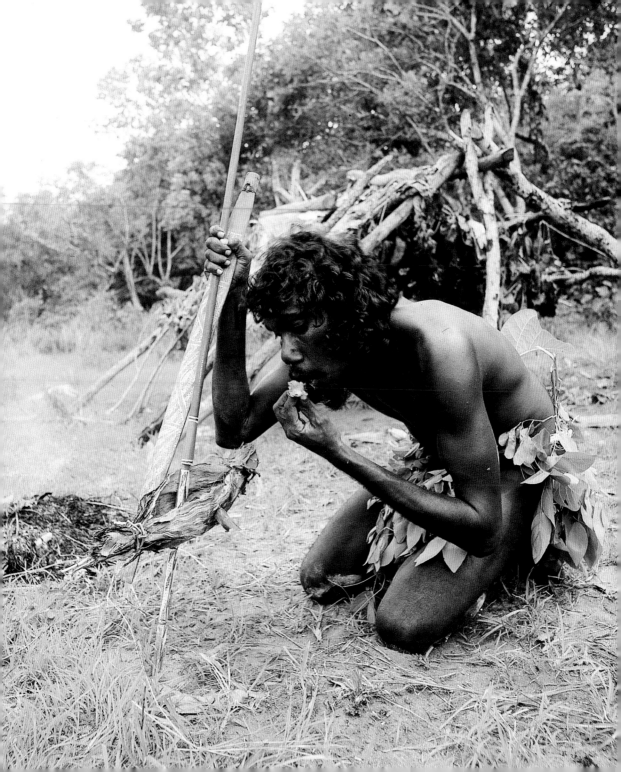

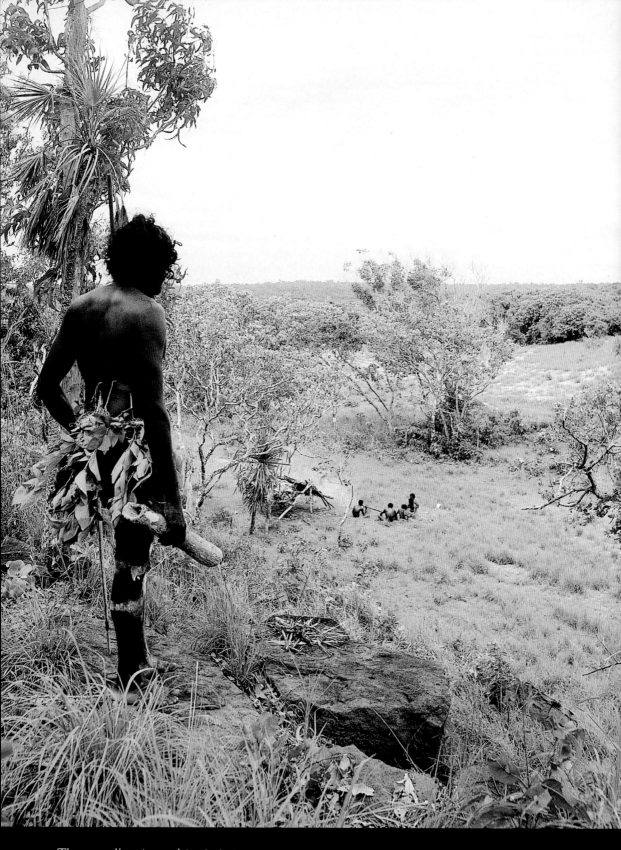

The raggalk spies on his victim's camp.
Illness, evil and misfortune are thought to be the surreptitious ploy of enemies.
A young actor shows how a spy visits a camp, planning some mischief,
while the owners are away, to plan his pay-back.

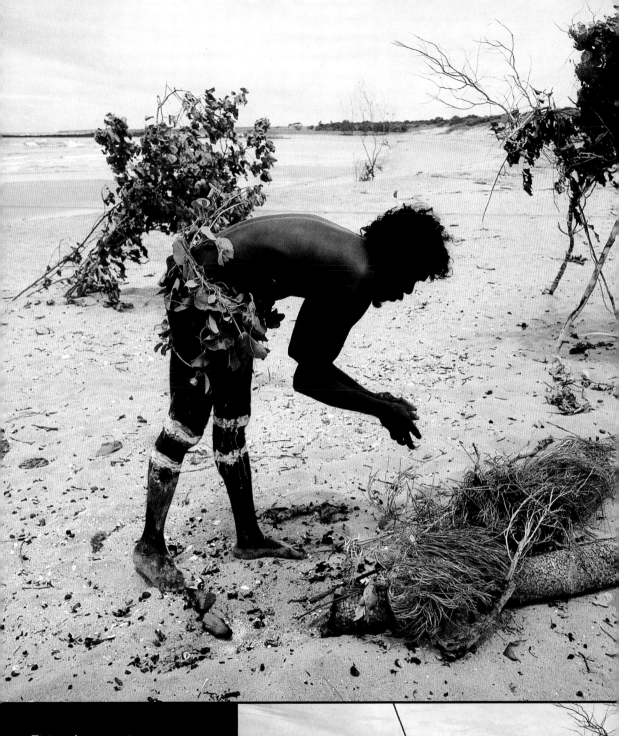

Firing the campsite.
The galka finds that a bowel
has been emptied near a
deserted camp.
He piles inflammable brush
over it between two logs and
sets it on fire.
Burning the excreta is
designed to produce
abdominal pain and
runny bowels.

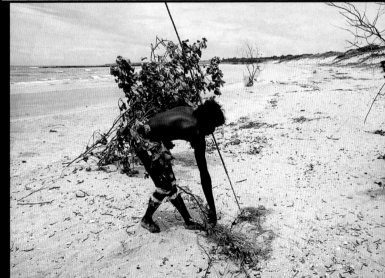

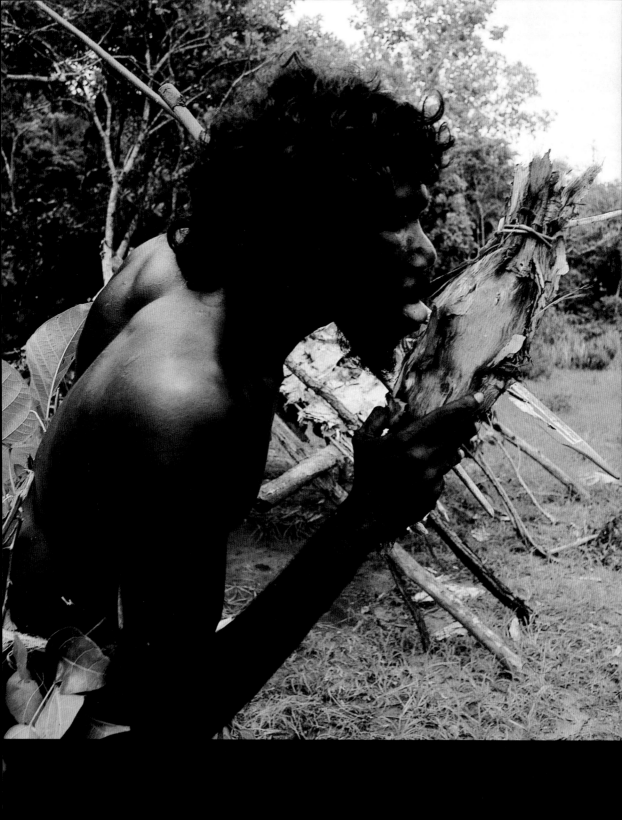

A galka spears the cup.
We are shown how the sinister intruder perforates the cup with his spear.
This is considered the cause of ulcers around the mouth and lips,
or the sore shiny bright red tongue prevalent where food is scarce.

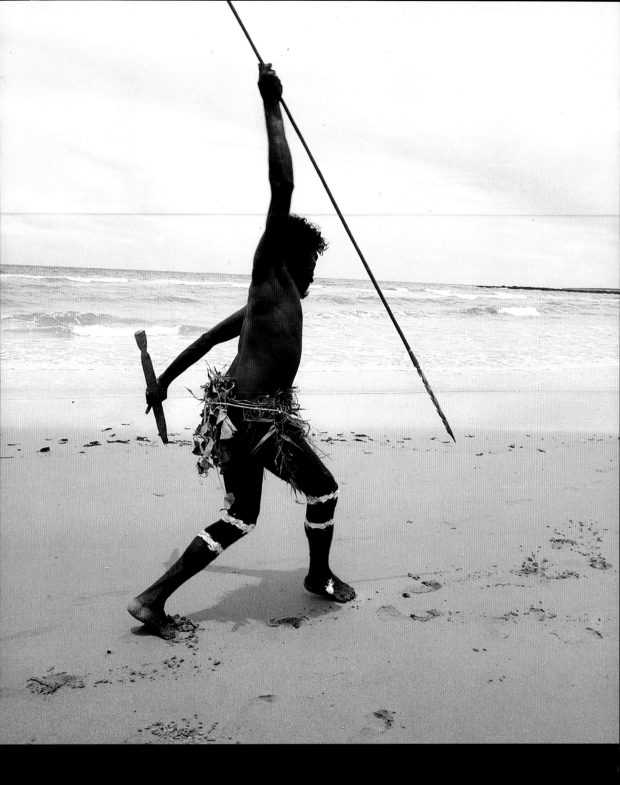

Spearing the wet patch on the sand.
This galka shows no mercy to a urine patch that he has discovered on the sand of the beach above the tide mark.
Scalding voiding is common among the women of these camps; one need look no further for the cause.
Always conceal the urine patch!

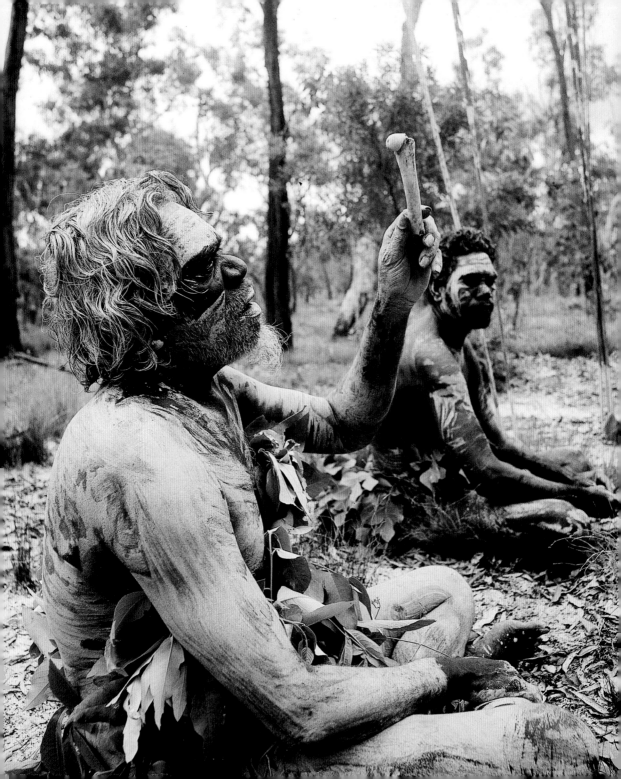

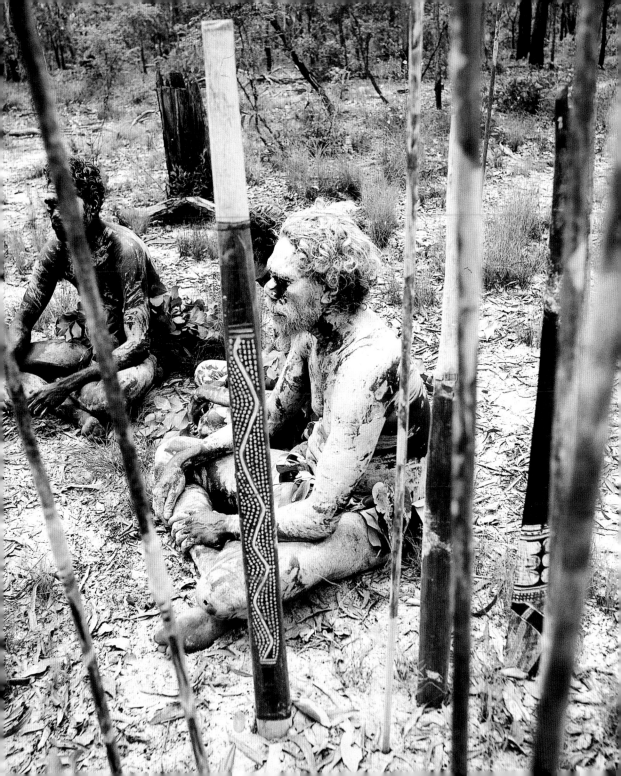

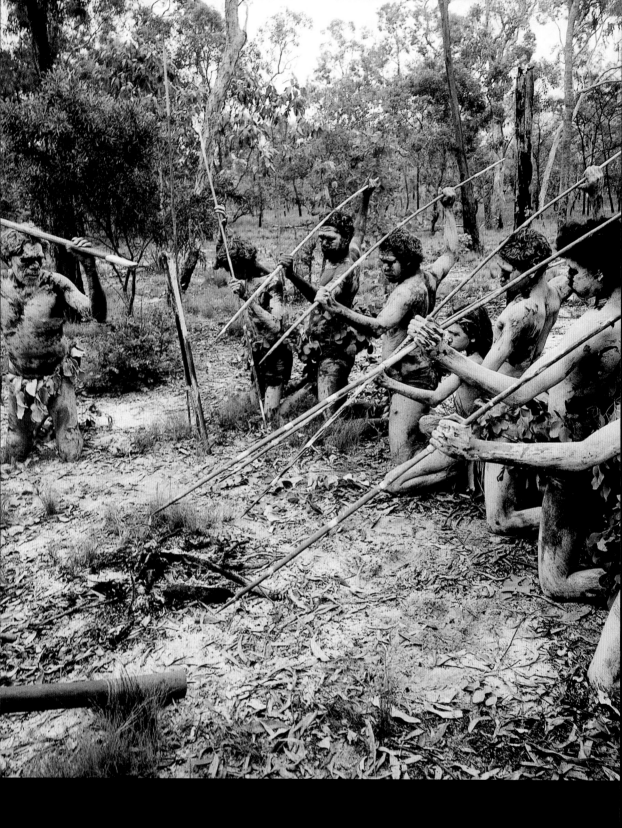

Pointing the ashes.
The clan group, including the younger men, direct the tips of their spears
toward a fire on the ground where the relics of their enemy are being burned.
They sing to his death.

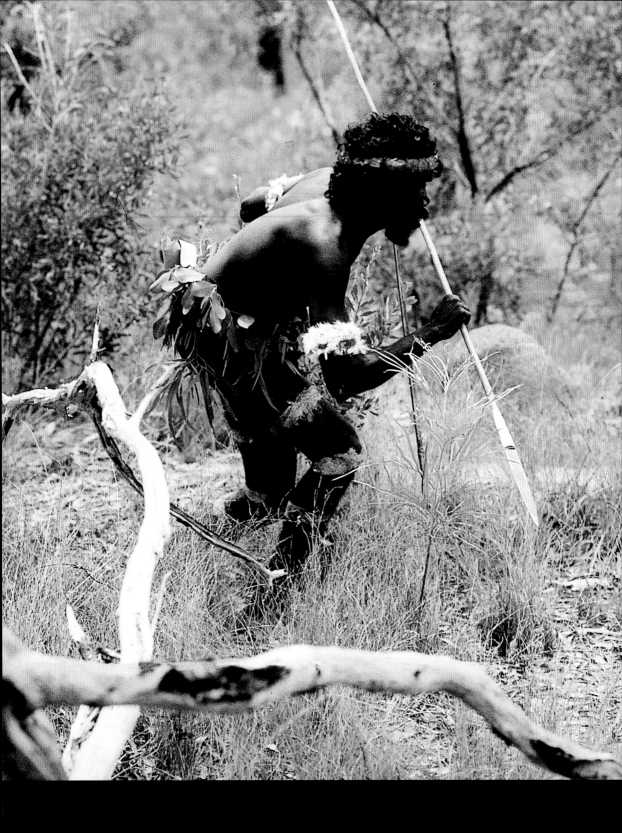

The flight of the galka.
Word now reaches the galka, perhaps through the calls of birds, that the angry clan is in hot pursuit. He sneaks furtively through the undergrowth, hoping to elude those who trail his steps.

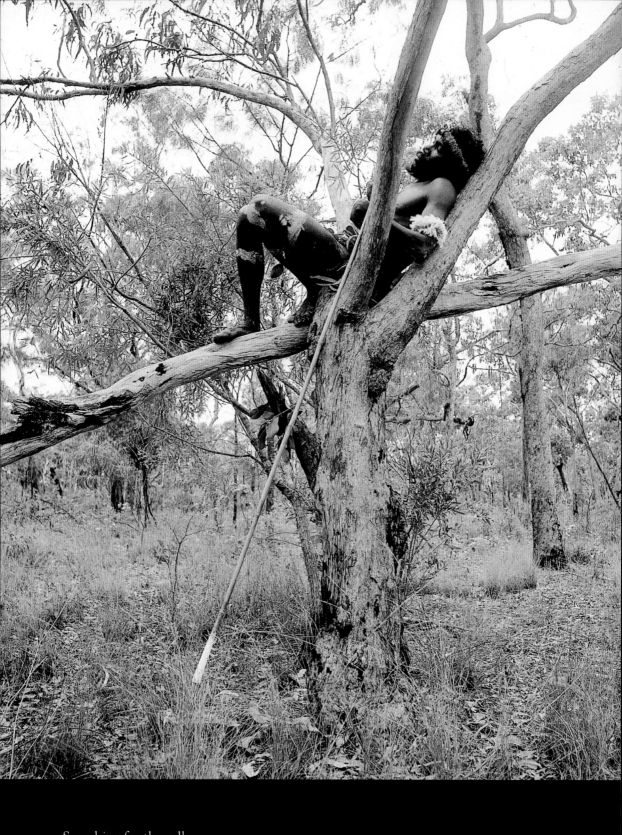

Searching for the galka.
It is hard to track down the evil agent of sickness because of
his refusal to reveal signs of a camp.
Thus he sleeps aloft in trees, resting the tip of his spear
on the ground. Our actor shows how it must appear.

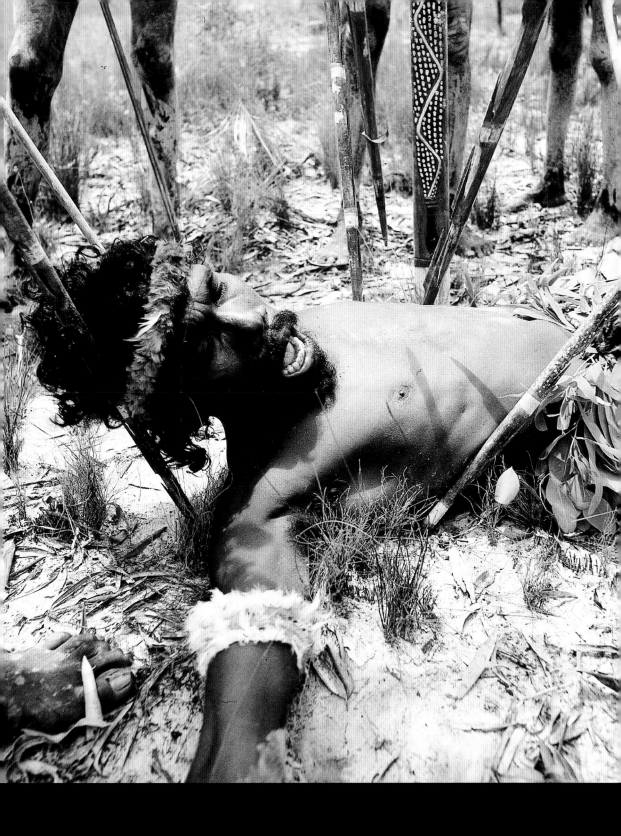

The galka is overtaken.
Justice prevails! A whistling spear brings down the galka in his flight.
Pursuers will have time to overtake him and wreak their pay-back for all his hurts and
harms inflicted upon their people. Now they can live in peace and health.

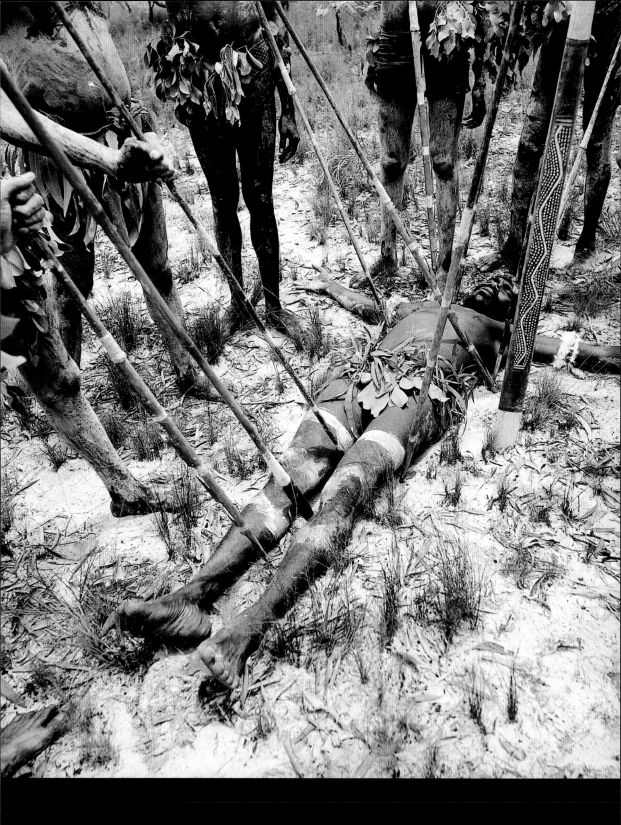

The galka is destroyed.
Supine on the ground, and surrounded by the pursuing clan, the galka meets his end.
The actor demonstrating this fate seems not unaware of the imagery of the crucifixion of
Christ. He is slaughtered. They are redeemed and restored.
So runs the saga of sickness.

the algae and are in turn eaten by big fish, which the men catch. As a disease, ciguatera poisoning is on the increase.

In an endemic ciguatera zone, some people suggest that you should first try out a piece of your big catch on the cat. Most people are not prepared to wait out the time needed for this test: they like to eat their fish as fresh as possible. Some brave fishermen try out a very small taste before making a meal of it, but this is dangerous. My friend Douglass Baglin had a serious attack of ciguatera on his yacht while cruising the Pacific. He and fellow members of the crew, hardly able to breathe, just managed to creep into Pearl Harbor in Hawaii. They were laid up for a month in the Queen's Hospital in Honolulu, grateful to God to survive.

'Why didn't you try that fish first on the ship's cat?' I asked Douglass.

'We didn't have a ship's cat.'

'What, put to sea on the Pacific without a ship's cat? Why, the cat is the most important member of the crew. Matthew Flinders had a cat on the *Investigator* which he called Trim. He wrote a book about Trim for children to read.'

'He never used Trim as a guinea pig,' retorted Douglass. 'Nor would I!'

'You'll have to do better,' I told him. 'Some people think that puffer fish are the deadliest. But only a fool would eat puffer fish! Ciguatera fish look so beautiful that you forget the risk—like those girls in Honolulu you met as soon as you were feeling better.'

This was badinage, of course: the conventional kidding of old buddies. But behind all that, we shared a deep concern for the Pacific and what would become of it. We believed that in fifteen or twenty years it would be the Pacific's turn, in the march of history, to become the world's great economic zone. And we doubted that the ASEAN, Asian and Pacific-rim Western countries would act in any cooperative fashion. That had become clear enough in the various exercises in which both of us had engaged to promote this end. Ciguatera poisoning seemed a symptom, a sinister signal of malaise to come. Perhaps the Pacific nations could come together in the first place over this dire challenge—as we saw it—to their food supply?

Dr Tilman Ruff is an infectious disease physician in Melbourne. His paper in the *Lancet*, 28 January 1989, shows evidence that the incidence of this disease in the Pacific Ocean is related to military activities that disturb coral reef ecology. Nuclear test explosions and their infrastructure are the major components of such military activity, Dr Ruff believes.

From the point of view of this book, ciguatera poisoning is of particular interest in that the Yolngu do not blame sorcery for it. They know *gunampi* well enough, but they put it down to a sickness of coral fish that are feeding on dead coral. They would strongly support Dr Tilman Ruff's conclusion.

1 Chaseling W (1957) *Yulengor* The Epworth Press London.

2 Wells E (1982) *Reward and Punishment in Arnhem Land 1962-1963* Australian Institute of Aboriginal Studies Canberra.

3 Ferdinand Magellan (1480–1521), Portuguese navigator, reached the coast of South America in 1519 and navigated the strait that now bears his name. He was killed in the Philippines, but one of his ships returned to Spain in 1522, and so was the first to circumnavigate the globe.

4 This is the author's English spelling of the Gupapuyngu word Ngulwado, or coral.

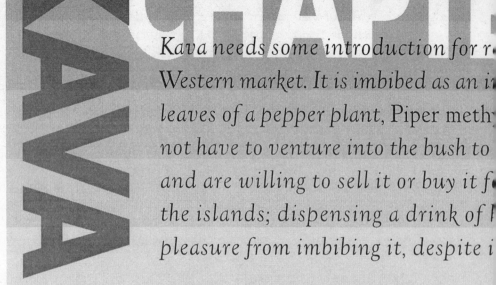

Kava needs some introduction for r
Western market. It is imbibed as an i
leaves of a pepper plant, Piper methy
not have to venture into the bush to
and are willing to sell it or buy it f
the islands; dispensing a drink of l
pleasure from imbibing it, despite i

the church

The categorization of kava as a narcotic follows the standard usage of this term for a substance that blunts the senses, relieves pain, lowers consciousness to the point of mild clouding and eventually induces sleep. This refers to its modest consumption; massive consumption produces complete insensibility. Habitual consumption of large amounts soon brings general ill-health in which scaling of the skin is the most obvious feature. Polynesians look upon kava as a gift qualified by pros and cons, depending on dosage and manner of preparation.

Since the plant *Piper methysticum* is peculiar to the South Sea islands, why should its use be discussed in a text devoted to the exotic diseases of Arnhem Landers? The plant does not grow in Australia. Were quantities of kava exported across the

...ers acquainted only with the dangerous drugs on the

...xicating narcotic beverage, prepared from the roots or

...cum, growing in the South Pacific islands. Polynesians do

...ect the wild plant. They cultivate it as a crop in their gardens

...oney. Its use is widespread, being part of the social fabric of

...u is an expression of hospitality. Many certainly derive

...uestionable taste.

drink

Pacific Ocean and the Coral Sea to confuse the already harassed Arnhem Landers confronted by modernity in the 'top end' of Australia? This is precisely what happened, in the early 1980s, with the assistance of Christian ministers.

Arnhem Landers were introduced to kava by missionaries who came to the settlement at Yirrkala from Fiji, Tonga and outlying Christianised countries. These visitors exerted great influence. Shocked by the disastrous effects of alcohol among Aboriginal groups, a number of them recommended kava in preference. They invited leading Arnhem Land people to visit Polynesia, where the kava ceremony deeply impressed them. The Polynesians' socially integrated moderate consumption of kava was infinitely preferable to the Arnhem Landers who thought: If only our people had a drug of this kind, which did not provoke its consumers to fight and to fornicate! On the contrary, kava drinkers in the South Seas seemed to talk in a sociable way, then dropped off to sleep!

At the introduction of kava to Arnhem Land the general view was that it brought happy pros, and no cons. Was it the solution to that bugbear of indigenous Australians, the demon drink? I discussed kava with a number of Arnhem Landers whom I had known for many years. Our talks were detailed, conducted in English or in a mixture of Aboriginal English and Yolngu vernacular. They well describe the development of the kava craze and the early assessment of its pros and cons. Names are coded, as in Cawte, 1986.

TR, the chairman of the Town Council, a capable and responsible man in early middle age, is the main importer and purveyor of kava for this community. He said that the Tongan variety is more popular than the Fijian: it is whiter and stronger in action than the darker Fijian powder. Perhaps it is dried better before it is powdered. He sells it at 15 dollars a packet and says he is not interested in making a profit. His motive is to challenge alcohol: if there were no kava, people would be constantly flying out of the dry community 'on business' to get alcohol and smuggling it home again. He expressed some surprise at how widespread kava is becoming, and how it pushes the craving for drink out of many people's minds. He describes it as an experiment and he is waiting to see how it will turn out. Yolngu often become enthusiastic about something new, only to let it lapse later; perhaps kava is only a craze and will die away? His own ambition in life is to start a fishery so that the people's diet will be better. He is buying nets and will start a business after his term as chairman of the Council. Perhaps in time they might rebuild the fish packing and freezing works which the missionaries had started. He then sold me a packet of kava.

IF, a former chairman of the Council, is widely respected for his experience and judgment. He had been to Fiji many years before and approved of kava there, because only one drink is taken and that in a ceremony. But here it is the same as drinking beer in a pub, except that sessions last 24 hours or more, and there is no doubt that drinkers become drunk. He has come to the view that kava is most unfortunate for the community. He said that the family is no good any more: parents are away for too long and the children are not looked after. Steady drinkers become tired and give no thought to food or preparing meals

for themselves or the family. Kava drinkers are not violent, but they are selfish. He does not feel kava is a passing fad: he predicts that it will grow and have even more serious effects. He explained the distribution more clearly. The Tongan kava, which makes you more drunk, is shipped to a Tongan agent in Sydney who places it into plastic bags which he packs into smaller boxes and mails direct to Yirrkala and Elcho Island, from where it is flown to the homeland centres. The Fijian kava is handled by a dealer in Darwin. He is convinced that the handlers are making a good profit, and he nominated a large sum of money. He worries about the solution to the problem. If he had the power he would ration it. Each person would then only get a limited quantity of kava a day. (It is of interest that this informant has himself given up smoking because of chest disease, and seems to have cured his son of petrol sniffing.)

LF is one of the leading health workers. He said that lots of Balanda (derived from 'Hollander', the Macassan word for white man) criticize kava but he sees its good side. People drinking kava talk, sing and tell stories all night, but they are good stories, and they talk about jobs and make plans for the future. That is quite different from drinking liquor, which makes people remember old grudges and clan fighting. People who are lonely, or shamed, come into the circle and share in the talk. His understanding is that in Samoa and Fiji kava is used to welcome strangers and to make friendships. He pointed out that in Australia it is perfectly legal: it goes through Australian Customs and Quarantine, who approve of it. He himself uses it; when he is tired, three or four cups relax him. He stopped indulging for a while, because of the Balanda criticisms, but has taken it up again. Sometimes Yolngu use it for special ceremonies, such as when the new minister was ordained. He encourages people to drink it with milk beside them, and he stresses hygiene: those who mix it in the aluminium bowl should have clean hands, with no sores on their skin. He feels that petrol sniffing is less avidly pursued by children because of kava, and it keeps the homeland centre people happy, so that they go away less to get alcohol. In short, he said it is very good for Yolngu because it brings the people together in peace. The Tongan and Fijian missionaries at Yirrkala are teaching the people to combine it with due ceremonial.

JZ is a notable bark painter, who teaches the art in school; he is also an active member of the church. He calls kava the 'church drink' and he feels that the church says nothing against it. He thinks it has the same energy as 'pot'. It can turn the mind anywhere, but it can bring on a fiery stage—and he has learned to stop before that! Once he saw visions from it, and could not make out what they were. He does not want visions coming from outside, from kava; they will not be true ones. He can often see visions of the sacred designs (rangga) in his mind, in his meditation rather than his dream. Truly sacred designs come into his mind to settle an argument about rangga. He does not want any help from kava: he wants his visions to come in pure messages from the Yolngu ancestors, and so he never mixes up kava with his Yolngu life.

FD is a distinguished elder who helped Reverend W Chaseling to establish the mission at Yirrkala before the war. He regards himself, and is regarded by others, as an authority of Yolngu law. He said that kava is not as dangerous as alcohol, but it seems to make the people who drink a lot of it grow older and blacker. 'They look like old, black men!' He thinks harm comes to them because kava makes them lazy and they don't eat enough animal and vegetable food. It also costs a lot—but there is plenty of money about to pay for it, so that cost does not matter much. It is all right in Fiji because they have a strong law governing it, to use it for special meetings, controlled by the chief, and as a welcome drink for important visitors. The law in Fiji is that the people who are invited to the kava meetings must take a shower and clean up, like going to church. But here we have no law at all. People drink it to get drunk. The Fiji Methodists sent it to the Methodists in Australia. He considered that the church are the people behind it—or they were behind it in the beginning.

UY is my clan 'brother', and he called

on me to share a cup of coffee. After we parted, he came back to ask for 30 dollars. 'Lend me 30 dollars for two packets of kava for tonight.' He said that five cups made him feel happy, rather like being drunk; after 10 cups he could no longer talk and then fell asleep. I 'lent' him 15 dollars because he is my 'brother', and I asked him to make me a certain carving of one of the clan ancestors in whom I am interested, and to take the loan off the price. He agreed with alacrity. I formed the impression while talking to him that he is psychologically dependent upon kava and wants it most nights. Without it, nights are dull and wearisome for him.

RE was formerly the gardener but is now in a job encouraging people at homeland centres to grow bananas and pawpaw. He too reported that the Tongan form of kava is preferred over the Fijian because it makes people drunker quicker. He does not think the plant can be grown locally because the soil is wrong. He emphasized the advantages of kava over liquor: when people get drunk on kava they feel happy, like to talk and sing the manikay or traditional songs. They do not fight or chase after women. They just sit down and when drunk enough they go off to sleep. The gambling craze has also died down because of kava, although when people run out of money for kava, they play cards for it. The drawbacks of kava have to do with health—the falling off in energy makes it easy to spot those who take too much kava and the fatigue often stops them coming to work. But all the northern Yolngu towns are using it, and in most places it is displacing alcohol. His wife confirmed what he said.

In this community there is a small number of psychotic people, in whom I have taken a special interest. They are not easy to treat, being considerably isolated socially, often teased by children, and poorly if at all compliant with medications. A Yolngu health worker told me of one psychotic individual who, he said, has 'come closer' to the people since kava was introduced. This patient is now a moderate though fairly regular kava consumer. In response to my question, my informant could not decide whether the kava has improved this patient's disposition, or whether the community is more accepting of him and his strange thinking.

On this visit I was able to see three other schizophrenics. One suffers from a disorder in which he is erratic and unpredictable, sometimes showing a fatuous and grandiose manner. He has heard voices whispering to him for about ten years, and he becomes suspicious, lurking much of the time inside his house. Since his speech is often hard to follow he is ridiculed a good deal by his children, who mimic him. When I saw him on this occasion I found him more relaxed, rational and conversational. He said his mind is 'free' and the voices are not bothering him. He can now mix with strangers, something he would never do before. He has been taking kava several nights a week for about a year, especially when he feels 'uptight'. He is welcomed by the rings of kava drinkers, including young men with whom he did not previously consort. He has found a new social life with them; he said he mostly talked about the gospel and joined in the singing.

I saw a chronic schizophrenic older man, whose conversation is so garbled that I have never been able to understand it. He is almost completely socially alienated, lives alone and wanders the town by himself. For years I have seen him tramping the roads as if he were going somewhere, muttering to himself and with an angry unapproachable demeanour. On this occasion he was more affable and I had the longest exchange ever with him; although his conversation still sounded like a 'word salad', his mood was amiable. I heard from the health worker that he too was accepted now at the kava rings. 'People who are lonely or shamed come into the circle and share the talk.'

A third psychotic had a prolonged social withdrawal for which he declined antidepressant medication or other help from the health centre. He was inactive, slow of speech and for much of the time shut himself in his house. His wife attended him closely and he would not permit her out of his sight. I was unsure of his diagnosis, especially as his elder sister has a 20-year history of severe schizophrenia, made more manageable by fluphenazine injections. On the present visit I learned that he now joins the kava rings and is generally considered to be much improved.

In the five years after these conversations were recorded, I followed the trajectory of kava consumption with mounting disbelief. To avoid confusion, this intake of kava should be designated as massive, rather than as mild or even moderate. The Arnhem Landers turned kava into an exotic disease!

Those who may have advocated the supply of kava to Arnhem Landers as a substitute for alcohol did not know the potency of kava, or the latency of Aboriginal people for excess—and for exotic disease. The Arnhem Landers, sitting under trees around kava bowls or buckets for many hours, might consume up to a hundred times the quantity normally imbibed in the Pacific Islands.

Notwithstanding the employment of the right social trappings—the large aluminium mixing bowl or bucket in the centre of the ring, and the coconut shell passing from hand to hand—the drinking of kava in Arnhem Land bore the imprint of Arnhem Land temperament. A session might last for 24 hours and be repeated several times a week. The kava rings were not composed along the traditional authoritarian clan or moiety lines, as in the religious ceremonials or *bungguls*. They were distinctly secular.

The first effect noticed by a kava drinker is numbing of the mouth—a sensation that led some partakers to suggest that it might make a good dental anaesthetic! The sensation might spoil the appetite. The early effects are not unlike those of a minor tranquilliser. Drinkers relax, talk amiably and join in the singing of songs old and new, until such time as the sedative effect predominates and they drop off to sleep where they sit. At least a part of the eventual sedative effect arises from fatigue and sleep deprivation. Unlike alcohol effects in the same groups, users do not revive old grievances and are not prone to act upon aggressive or sexual impulses.

Loss of weight commonly occurs after steady use of kava. Heavy habitues show a strong trend to repeat the session after a day or two, suggesting either psychological or physiological dependence, or both.

Symptoms were immediately recognized by nurses and health workers at the sick bay. Lassitude and apathy were common, often ascribed to loss of sleep. There was a high absenteeism from work. A teacher told me that children fall asleep in her morning class and give the reason as kava. She likened its effect to that of smoking 'pot'. The detachment and drowsiness, with the child's head on the desk, identified the partakers.

A common physical sign was the darkening of exposed skin, sometimes accompanied by a scaliness, which gave the patient the appearance of having aged. It could proceed to exfoliative dermatitis, including loss of hair and eyebrows falling out. Occasionally there were allergic reactions with running eyes and noses. Puffy skin could close the eyes entirely. One nurse told me of heavy users who showed elevation of blood pressure and complaints of chest pain. Some individuals described visions and nightmares. The nurse suspected that most people so affected do not report to the clinic, sleeping off the effects at home. Several of the more

seriously affected had to be flown out to the district hospital more than a hundred miles away on the medical plane. After recuperating in hospital, they hastened to join a band of local people drinking alcohol in the bed of the creek below the hotel. A belief arose that alcohol is the cure for the bad effects of kava! A further belief then became current that kava and alcohol have counteracting effects and should be drunk together, or one after the other. This is the custom in Sydney hotels, where Polynesians or Aboriginal people imbibe: a drink of kava is followed by a beer chaser.

The use and misuse of kava in Northern Australia naturally aroused academic interest. A monograph on this subject was published in 1982.[2] It includes many recent observations. My Australian findings are linked with those of psychologist Robert J Gregory on Oceania, under the title 'The Principle of Alien Poisons'. They are sufficiently concise to form a useful summary for this chapter, without unduly repeating what has been covered before.

I observed the increasing role of kava from the early 1980s in a community in Northeast Arnhem Land. I had visited this community regularly for nearly 20 years, when people were quite abstinent, through the period when people were becoming used to the self-regulating consumption of alcohol. The official reason for my continued visits was to offer my services as a medical practitioner and psychiatrist, but my private interest, encouraged by them, lay in their healing, art, poetry, religion and ceremonial, not to mention the social power system, fading before the advent of modern times. They had not yielded up their practice of polygyny.

Kava arrived without its usual philosophy. Crates were shipped from its Pacific sources containing plastic packages of dried root weighing 500 each, 'enough for one or two sessions', sold at $15. The people knew that the beverage was to be consumed from coconut husks while sitting in circles under trees. It had been suggested by visiting ministers from Fiji that kava might replace alcohol, and quell the quarrels stirred by alcohol indulgence. No taboos were applied. It was drunk 'democratically' by men, women and children. Feasts were hardly possible. The people were mainly hungry for a strong pharmacological effect to replace that of alcohol. Vast dosages were consumed at some sessions. Any resemblance with Pacific Island scene or ceremonies was correspondingly diluted.

Importers and (white) agents were doubtless encouraged by the sales and the profits. They made sanctimonious justifications about their worthy aims of replacing alcohol. It was easy for adventurers to rationalize the importation of kava, particularly as it was classified as a 'food product' in its importation through the Customs Department.

Unlike the Pacific communities, nobody attempted to grow the pepper bush, though the climate may have been favourable. Payment through social service provisions and pensions seemed satisfactory to most of the consumers. About half the men in this community adopted its use to varying degrees; about half declined. It was my observation that kava users were in general 'other-directed' personalities, while non-users were inner-directed, to employ a distinction that was popularized by David Reisman in The Lonely Crowd (1973). Hence they were less open to fads. Non-users of kava were mostly of higher social status, too.

The widespread assumption that Aborigines are all 'other-directed' and of 'equal social status' produces misleading stereotypes that retard proper relations with them. The stereotype that all Aborigines are 'other-related' has the same drawback that it would in Western society. Assumptions like this lead to patterns of fraternity for the group, rather than an individual approach to the person.

This community comprised a warlike assembly of Arnhem Land clans that

were learning to live together in peace. Kava helped, so a typical grateful response was: 'When people get drunk on kava they feel happy. They like to talk or to sing the traditional songs. They do not want to fight or chase after women. They just sit down and when drunk enough they go off to sleep.'

The gambling craze also died down because of kava. However, when people ran out of money to pay for kava, they played cards for it.

The population of the new village, founded in 1943 at the time of Japanese bombing of this coastline, made up of some twelve warring clans from surrounding territories in Arnhem Land, lost its usual animation. In evaluating this, one had to remember that the traditional human ecology of Australian Aborigines tends to foster personality characteristics that distinguish them from the gardening cultures of Oceania. Unlike South Sea Islanders, Aborigines depend upon what nature sends them to eat and this blessing is irregular and seasonal.

At times of plenty Aborigines are usually busy and grow fat. At times of scarcity they are inactive and grow thin. This perennial association leads to a tendency to consume all that is at hand—whether it is food, alcohol or kava— without storing it for another day. This seems one of the conceptual problems in adapting to Western society. It resembles the Carpe Diem philosophy commended by the poet Horace—to gather the fruits of the day.

Aboriginal personality characteristics are not calculated to encourage modulated usage of drugs such as narcotic pepper (nor of alcohol, for that matter) over planned cycles of social or religious conduct, nor to consider growing the crop rather than importing it, at a high cost, paid by social services and pensions.

On the basis of these findings, heavy kava usage had to be regarded as very harmful to health. I recommended that steps should be taken to prevent its introduction into Aboriginal communities where it is not yet available, and that Customs should reconsider its classification as a 'food product'. I classified it as a poison.

An outstanding contrast is noted between the effect of kava in one of its sites of origin (described by Dr Gregory in the 1988 monograph already cited), the island of Tanna, Vanuatu, and secondarily on Elcho Island, Arnhem Land. This contrast merits attention for the light it sheds on the narcotic pepper, kava, the effects of which are clearly dependent on cultural factors determining usage. It affords a classic example of the law emphasized by the German toxicologist Gustav Schenk[3] that poisons and stimulants from abroad are far more deleterious than those of one's own country—the 'Law of Alien Poisons'.

Perhaps the most poignant comment on this new exotic disease in Arnhem Land is the one offered by Grayson Gerrard, an anthropologist, who contributed to the 1988 monograph a paper entitled: 'Use of Kava in Two Aboriginal Settlements'. She writes:

The pressures on this emerging society are of enormity, and the last comment I would like to make in this paper—and I do not intend it as a flippant one at all—is that if I myself were an Arnhem Lander today, I too would place mind-altering drugs at a premium in my emerging hierarchy of valuing.

1 Cawte J (1986) Parameters of kava used as a challenge to alcohol *Australian and New Zealand Journal of Psychiatry* 20 (70–76).
2 Prescott J and McCall G (eds) *Kava: Use and Abuse in Australia and the South Pacific* Monograph No 5 of the National Drug and Alcohol Research Centre University of New South Wales Sydney.
3 Schenk G (1956) *The Book of Poisons* Translated from the German *Das Buch Der Gifte* by Michael Bullock, Werdenfield and Nicolson, 7 Cork Street, London W1.

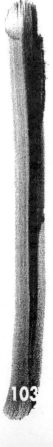

A plant of outstanding importance a
macrozamia. You can feast on it or it ca
comprise a single family, Cycadaceae
Cycadaceae, Zamiaceae and Stranger

# of wild

The name Burruwang palm is used for several species of *Macrozamia* palms in New South Wales. Some are called fool's pineapple. They have nothing to do with either palms or pineapples. The cycad palm in Arnhem Land is called *nartu* by the Yolngu, and it was the staple food from August to December, but without careful preparation the nut of the *nartu* is poisonous from its toxic component, cycasin. Its leaching can be treacherous and tricky.

After roasting them lightly to aid the removal of the husk from these walnut-sized nuts, Yolngu women crushed the seed, wrapped them in a paperbark parcel and then soaked them in a water-hole for five days to

food on these Arnhem Land savannahs was the cycad or
kill you. The order Cycadales was formerly thought to
but recent studies have distinguished three families,
aceae—the latter not occurring in Australia.

food

wash out the poison. Sometimes they let the mush ferment like dough. Sometimes they cut or crushed the nuts before soaking to assist the elution of the poison. Sometimes they baked them as dough, on fire-heated stones. The loaf might be sweetened by wild honey. It made a good damper.

Early European explorers who tried to survive on bush food became sick: either dismally constipated or running the bloody flux, when not vomiting. Amazing men! The diary of the Prussian naturalist and explorer Ludwig Leichhardt (1813–1848)[1] makes observations on cycad seeds and their preparation by the residents by cutting, elution in water and subsequent fermentation in bags.

Ludwig Leichhardt's memoir on cycad seeds (page 406 of his journal) deserves to be revived; he became an expert on the treachery of Australian food. He wrote:

As we passed the cycas groves, some of the dry fruit was found and tasted by several of my companions, upon whom it acted like a strong emetic, resembling in this particular the fruit of Zamia spiralis, (R. Br.) of New South Wales. The natives, at this season, seemed to live principally on the seeds of Pandanus spiralis, (R.Br.) and Cycas; but both evidently required much preparation to destroy their deleterious properties.

I also observed that seeds of cycas were cut into very thin slices, about the size of a shilling, and these were spread out carefully on the ground to dry, after which, (as I saw in another camp a few days later) it seemed that the dry slices are put for several days in water, and, after a good soaking, are closely tied up in tea-tree bark to undergo a peculiar process of fermentation.

We found here the carcase of a crocodile; and the skull of another was found near our camp at Cycas Creek. After crossing the river, we followed down its left bank to the lower ford, in order to find some fresh water, and at last came to a small tea-tree gully with two pools of water, near which some natives were encamped; there were, however, only two very old men in the camp at the time, who, on seeing us, began to chant theirincantations. We were too anxious to examine the water to stand upon ceremony, and, when they saw us approach, they retired across the river to their friends, who were probably occupied at no great distance in collecting the seeds of pandanus and cycas. In the camp, we observed cycas seeds sliced and drying on the ground; and some pandanus seeds soaking in large vessels; emu bones were lying in the ashes, and the feet of the emu were rolled up and concealed between the tea-tree bark of the hut. A small packet contained red ochre to colour their bodies, and larger packets contained soaked cycas seeds, which seemed to be undergoing fermentation. They were of a mealy substance, and harmless; but had a musty taste and smell, resembling that of the common German cheese.

Cycad or *nartu* is plentiful, being the typical understorey of the eucalypt stringybark forests of Arnhem Land. Palatable and easily gathered, it was food of some popularity with or without the attraction of fermentation.

'What do you do if somebody is poisoned from eating *nartu*?' I asked Stingray Spine. We were looking at the graceful fronds of a fine specimen.

'I nearly died once at Milingimbi, from eating *nartu*,' he told me and recounted his experience.

Four of us young fellows, including Sea Water [Jim] here, were walking around

the countryside looking for a girl, maybe, and we came upon a dry billabong. In it was a well where the women were soaking bundles of nartu, wrapped up in paperbark. We were hungry so we stole some of it. One of us got into the well and unwrapped the paperbark. Two of us made a fire, and we baked it like damper for three hours, really cooked it. But the women must have put it in the water the previous day, because when we ate it we soon found the poison was still active.

Fifteen minutes after we ate it, my head started to spin. How do you feel? I asked Sea Water—My head is spinning! And you? Same way. And you? Same way. We ate it at the wrong time, too early. Soon we were vomiting, and our bowels were running, and our urine was running. I suppose we were lucky to have near us three remedies to cast out that poison from our bodies.

Soon after the vomiting started, I turned to look for a pandanus palm. The leaf and root of the pandanus is the only cure for the nartu. My mother and father had told me: get the white stuff from the base of the root. So we found the root of the pandanus and ate it and the vomiting ceased. The goodness of the pandanus ran from belly to head. We slept, and next morning we could not wake up, sleepy and drowsy till midday.

Another good cure is right here growing on the tree like an orchid. We call it djalkurrk.

[He indicated the bracket orchid growing on a tree trunk, Dendrobium dicuphum.] The juice in the stem is very sticky. It is useful for sticking the paint on bark paintings, or on the belly of dead or alive people we are painting. But it is also good for sores. It will keep the edges of a gaping wound stuck together, instead of a bandage, so that it heals quickly. Not like a bandage—more like plastic skin.

This big scar on my elbow was caused when I fell on some slippery weed on a reef and cut my arm on an oyster shell. It bled like running water. I looked for djalkurrk to mend my cut. I got some from an old man and the cut healed.

The best cures and medicine usually come

from sea. Rotten seaweed is good for massage. That's why I look so young. The seaweed and the crayfish is the proper power to defend me and my family. The flowers and roots of trees are all right, but the oceanic mixture is the cure.

If you doctors understood how we Warramirri Yolngu from Dhuldji and the thirty-four islands developed out of the sea, you would know that saltwater medicine is right for us when we are weak and out of sorts. You have to understand our genesis from Nulwardo, the coral god, to Rambila the squid god, then through several stages of Manda the octopus god, before we became, through the power of Marryalyan the sea-changer, the Warramirri men we are today.

For nine months this year I was feeling out of sorts and the only help I had for my feeling condition came from the ocean: oysters, turtle, fish, crayfish—just so long as it was from the salt water.

Just as there are two kinds of water, there are two kinds of food and two kinds of animal and two kinds of man. The feeling condition of the man depends on the mixture of the food. The mixture must be higher in salt water for the islander than for the inlander. It is risky for us Warramirri to live on the inland food.

You remember that ambergris from the stomach of the whale which we found when you and I walked on the beach at Cape Wessel? I mixed that with clamshell, and I rubbed a little on my head, like soap. That is what makes me look so young. Just a little. Not too much, or ten young ladies will be chasing us! And speaking of that, be careful not to take too many baths.

Stingray Spine is a fastidious man by any reasonable standards. In most of the houses at the township there are not the bathrooms, clean water, or hot water that encourage people to take a daily shower with soap. Consequently he suffers like all the other Yolngu from boils and other skin sores. But he has some compelling reasons why it is unwise and even unsafe to bathe the skin too much. He explained:

Most Balanda, and a lot of Yolngu want to keep clean all the time, day after day, because they think it's the gateway for the entry of the woman. Smelling nice makes sure the young woman will come to you. Bathe, cut your hair, shave, put a little whale oil on your face and head— that's what draws the mielk's [woman's] heart to the dirrimu [man]. That's why so many Yolngu and Balanda are keeping themselves clean all the time, hoping.

It's particularly dangerous to use too much whale oil. A man could easily have six women and they'll fight each other with jealousy. This forces everyone into trouble. I use only a little bit, just enough to keep me awake. But I don't wash, because I might easily get six mielk. I only like to bathe when my body gets stiff and hard, maybe once a month.

Using whale oil, or anything else, to draw a mielk to you, or to keep her on all the time, is very wrong. If a man does that, our law says fine him: with sticks or spear, or make him pay back a turtle, or a woman, to the old men.

But if you do attract another woman and you can't help it, because the love magic is sending your marr [inclination] that way, you can divorce your wife. A Yolngu divorce is not like a Balanda divorce. It is not a divorce forever. The woman is just kicked off for a year to make room for the new one to come in. The law says that you can move out the first mielk for a while, but she must come back. If she says, No, Yaka, I won't go, the husband has to stay unhappy, because his marr has gone out to the new one.

Hair is a tricky business with us. Shaving your beard can be risky. But growing it too much can be risky. That time I was sick, for that nine months when I lost my marr, I had long hair and beard. I was thinking too much that I was a grey-haired old man, in charge of a lot of maraian [sacred songs]. In actual truth I'm really quite young to be the owner of maraian. But I grew hair like an old man, and people in other places in Arnhem Land grew jealous of me. They wanted to cut me down so they threw mud on me, for nine long months. I shaved the beard off the day you and I came back from Marchinba—remember? That was the start of my recovery, that restoring the sacred object. Something tells me something's still wrong in the air, so I'm not leaving home camp. Sydney or Canberra may be all right, but something tells me not to leave home camp to go around in Arnhem Land. It's still not safe for me to go round and about.

Bathing in the sea is quite a different matter from bathing in the bathroom: safer and better. You know how my head becomes clouded over when I stay in your house in Sydney, because the air is crowded with strange spirits? So I always ask you to take me to the beach, to Bondi, Coogee or Maroubra, where the spirits of the sea blow on me. They refresh my marr. Swimming in the surf at Coogee makes me feel better at once.

You need salt inside, as well as outside, to keep you fresh. In 1962 a man came from New Guinea to teach us about elections, and the government called us in to Darwin to learn all about it. But I found it hard to think; my mind was blank. I failed the course. I couldn't find the words to answer the questions. The Returning Officer said to me: think about it tonight, and tell me in the morning. So I took a salt bath. I asked the cook in the kitchen for salt and I drank it. It strengthened me and let me think. I answered the six questions exactly right.

The islander like me who goes to the bush or the city gets lost and he loses his face for a few days or a week. Sea food is the cure, because its spirit refreshes our spirit. Turtle meat, seagull eggs, oysters, stingray—all sea creatures let you live life, enjoying the power and goodness of this life.

Reader, if Stingray Spine comes to stay in your home, or maybe one of his clansmen or women, please have oysters, prawns and fish in your refrigerator. Don't let him tyrannize you. On one occasion at my place, Stingray Spine spent hours pressing the liquid from kelp he gathered from Coogee beach, and he had me running around trying to find an octopus to put with it. I told him we weren't compiling a cook book.

'What is the antidote to the deadly sea wasp?' I really wanted him to tell me.

'Yaka Marngi,' he stopped talking. 'I don't know. The sea takes life away, if it wants to, and you cannot do a thing to stop it.'

Speaking of antidotes, there were months when Stingray Spine was so morose and retarded, so overclouded in his feeling condition that he did not seem to be getting better. I tried to find an antidote to his depression from my own pharmacopoeia. Tranquillizers did not help, and the tricyclic antidepressants were not effective; they may have helped a little. Finally he responded very promptly to a drug called a monoamine oxidase inhibitor. Whether it caught him as he was beginning to recover or whether it really lifted him up, who can say? Stingray Spine is sure it helped, and it did no harm.

He is so grateful to this drug that I will tell you its trade name—*Parstelin*, from the Smith, Kline and French Company. Only doctors can prescribe it. Any doctor who uses it has to supervise it carefully, for under certain conditions it can be harmful. I am never one to disparage the pharmaceutical industry. I often wonder what the drug firms buy one half so precious as the goods they sell. I have learned, however, to detect a few pitfalls on a patient's path, which the patient does not see and in he falls! But for all my study of pharmacology, my knowledge scarcely rivals that of Stingray Spine on his wild antidotes.

Ethnobotany was not my specialty. I gained my awareness of wild antidotes and remedies in a random manner, depending on chance observations and exchanges. A reader who wants a systematic survey of Australian plants that may have medicinal uses should turn to a detailed book, *Australian Medicinal Plants*, by E V Lassak and T McCarthy.[2] Hundreds of plants are reviewed in this book in relation to uses reported by Aborigines or by European settlers. The book has had numerous reprints since first publication. The volume begins with a caution: 'The authors and publishers waive any responsibility for injuries to readers of this book resulting from the use of plants listed here. Scientifically, their real effects have yet to be determined.'

Probably the best account of herbal remedies in a single tribal territory is Dulcie Levitt's *Aboriginal Use of Plants on Groote Eylandt*.[3] Dulcie Levitt was a botanist who worked with the Church Missionary Society on Groote Eylandt, Northern Territory, studying the natural environment and the part it played in the indigenous culture. I too worked on Groote Eylandt so her work caught my attention. She classifies the plants from both the botanical and the functional point of view. A good idea of her remarkable disclosures may be gained from considering just one item from her formulary, that which concerns wounds:

Great care was taken when approaching someone who had been seriously injured. It was realised that if flies got onto a deep wound they could be dangerous, so a man's friends did not rush up to him if he was injured. They lit a smoky fire with the smoke blowing towards the injured man, then walked in the smoke as they approached him to make sure that they did not carry flies on their bodies. If they found themselves getting out of range of the smoke they lit another fire, and another, until the last fire was near the patient with the smoke blowing over him. This kept flies away while the wound was being treated.

The harmful effect of foreign matter in an injury was also understood, and care was taken that no small pieces of bark, grit or other solid material was in the liquid used for treating wounds.

COCKY APPLE, BUSH MANGO, WILD QUINCE (PLANCHONIA CAREYA), MUKUWARA

Prepared as for sores, the liquid was poured into the wound, taking care not to get any solid matter into it, and the wound was then strapped firmly after the edges were pressed together. Sometimes, the bark from Mukuwara roots was used as strapping, sometimes the inner bark of Mabanda (yellow hibiscus) was used. It was used flat, and not made into string first.

YELLOW HIBISCUS, YARL TREE (HIBISCUS TILIACEUS) MABANDA, MILYURRKWA

The outer bark from a young shoot was scraped off and the inner bark and sapwood were shredded into a shell; fresh or salt water was added, and the container was placed near a fire to heat. When ready, the liquid was poured into the wound, taking care not to let any solid matter flow in with the liquid. The wound was then strapped firmly with Mabanda bark.

WHITE SAND LILY (CRINUM ASIATICUM), WHITE BUSH LILY (CRINUM UNIFLORUM), ADIKALYUBA

This was prepared as for sores but only the liquid was poured into the wound. The crushed and soaked bulb was sometimes placed over the wound after it had been closed by pressing the edges together, and was strapped in place with Mabanda bark or bark from the roots of Mukuwara.

SALTWATER SPIKE RUSH (ELEOCHARIS DULCIS), MIKIRRA

This is a small rush growing in swamps subject to flooding by high tides during the wet season. It is the same type as that found in freshwater billabongs, but the freshwater ones were never used medicinally. A handful of the saltwater rush was gathered and soaked in sea water, and the liquid was poured into the wound. The stems, which are soft and hollow, were then plastered over the

injury. It stung, but healed. The plaster
stayed in place without bandaging,
and eventually dropped off as
the injury healed.

An Aboriginal woman, speared with a
lama (shovel-nosed spear) during a fight
when she was about 10 years old, was
treated by this method. The spear went
through her upper arm and into her side
just below the armpit, leaving a gaping
wound in which the lung could be seen.
Her mother got saltwater Mikirra, soaked
the stems in sea water in a baler shell,
and after it had soaked for some time,
poured the liquid into the wounds. It
stung. The stems of the plant were then
plastered over the injury in her side and
over the two holes in her arm where the
spear had entered and left. The treatment was carried out while she was
standing up. The wound healed without
further treatment. As no attempt had
been made to draw the edges of the
wound together, she now has an indent-
ed scar on either side of her arm, and a
deep hole under the armpit. However,
fully pigmented skin has grown over the
injury, even at the bottom of the hole.

Miss Levitt's monograph similarly
details the household remedies in the
instances of bites, bleeding, boils and
sores, constipation, coughs and colds,
diarrhoea and so forth.

These detailed treatments for
wounds were the common knowledge
of the people as a whole and of the
experienced older women in particular. These treatments are undoubtedly
useful in many instances and in others
are open to the same objections as are
their European counterparts, if I may
point them out. For example, a fresh
wound that is not sutured is not likely
to heal by the first intention; you have
to close it up quickly. A fracture that is
not splinted such that the points above
and below the break are immobilized is
not going to be stable; bony union is
unlikely. A fluid that is not sterile and
is instilled into the eye or ear may
bring infection. These are of course

objections that can be levelled against
household remedies the world over,
since the beginning of medicine.

Although the Australian flora is
still far from being adequately known
and even less is known of the native
herbal formulary, two developments
promise to be of real assistance to
those who wish to explore this field.
The first number of the comprehensive
Flora of Australia was published in
1981 by the Australian Government
Publishing Service, Canberra, planned
to be followed by at least fifty further
numbers, published over a twenty-year
period. It reached Number 54 in 1992.
This ambitious work is intended for
use by professional botanists and other
scientists, and by knowledgeable ama-
teurs and students requiring botanical
information. It includes all flowering
and non-flowering plants known to be
indigenous or naturalised in Australia
but excludes bacteria.

A second development of value to
those who wish to study Australian
medicinal plants was the establishment
of the National Botanic Gardens in
Canberra. At the foot of Black
Mountain in a magnificent panoramic
setting is an extensive arboretum of
native plants. Particularly exciting is
the Aboriginal Trail, a walk which
leads the visitor to hundreds of species
used for food or for medicine. Well
signposted, it gives the visitor a vivid
impression of the scope of this field.
Alas, it is a field that seems destined to
remain poorly explored since, every
year, excellent Aboriginal teachers and
informants are taking their knowledge
to the grave.

That is why I took care to find out
what I could about the wild antidotes
of Arnhem Land from my mentors on
Elcho Island over the years. We talked

on this subject whenever there was time: that is, when I was not tied up with patients or they with ceremonials. This did not leave much time! Still, I learned something. For most observers, the field of herbal remedies is particularly inviting because it tends to bypass the horror of sorcery. One can claim expertise in traditional healing by concentrating on bush remedies, overlooking the suspicion of curses.

Stingray Spine is not a patient teacher. He expects you to listen and remember it first time. He does not like to have to go over the same ground again. He becomes bored. But if I approach him on a subject I have been researching—such as this one—antidotes to cycad poisoning—he can always make it come alive with personal memories and illustrations.

Readers who lack tribal access, and friends such as Stingray Spine, are able to treasure on their bookshelves a monumental publication, *Bush Food: Aboriginal Food and Herbal Medicine.*[4] The volume is illustrated lavishly with specially commissioned colour photographs, as a compendium of the kinds of food eaten by Aborigines. It shows how food is caught or gathered, hunted or picked, how it is prepared and cooked, and what nutritional value it has. It also considers the use of natural products in traditional Aboriginal herbal medicine. The same author recently gave us a *Companion guide to Bush Food.*

An encyclopedia has been produced by the Aboriginal Community of the Northern Territory, entitled *Traditional Bush Medicine: An Aboriginal Pharmacopoeia.*[6] The botany is comprehensive and the colour photographs superb. Medical doctors may query the therapeutic uses attributed to the plants, which seem to be infinite in their actions. However, the encyclopedia includes at the start a small but salutary note:

> WE CAUTION
> THOSE WHO WOULD USE THIS TEXT AS A
> MANUAL OF MEDICAL TREATMENT.
> MANY OF THE SUBSTANCES ARE
> TOXIC AND CAN CAUSE
> DEATH OR BLINDNESS
> IF IMPROPERLY USED.

1 Leichhardt L (1847) *Journal of an Overland Expedition from Moreton Bay to Port Essington, a Distance of Upwards of 3000 Miles, during the years 1844–45* Original publication 1847 T & W Boone London (1980 Facsimile Doubleday, Lane Cove).

2 Lassak E V and McCarthy T (1983) *Australian Medicinal Plants* Metheun Australia (Reprinted 1984, 1985, 1987, 1990. Mandarin, of Octopus Publishing Group. Reprinted 1992).

3 Levitt D (1981) *Plants and People: Aboriginal Uses of Plants on Groote Eylandt* Australian Institute of Aboriginal Studies, Canberra.

4 Isaacs J (1987) *Bush Food: Aboriginal Food and Herbal Medicine* Weldons Pty Ltd, Sydney.

5 Isaacs J (1996) *A Companion Guide to Bush Food.* Lansdowne Publishing, Sydney.

6 *Traditional Bush Medicines: An Aboriginal Pharmacopoeia* (1988) From the Aboriginal Communities of the Northern Territory of Australia, Greenhouse Publications, Richmond Victoria.

Readers of this book will be prepared
at the Mission after World War II and
They were spellbound at the profusion
packaged conveniently and seemed to

# of whit

Furthermore, there was tobacco, for which they all
longed, on the shelves with the flour and sugar.
How easy life would be!Before long they began
to lose their health, never to regain the energy
that invigorated them while they fed themselves out in the bush. A charge could
now be levelled that the flour and sugar,
so white and immaculate, were in subtle ways more treacherous than the
starch from cycads. Here is the tale
of a stalwart man affected by this
new exotic ill that I call saccharine disease. His lost manhood
was not due to sorcery.

The totemic owners of
Marrna the shark in the
Dardiwuy clan depict it
on their bark paintings.
The sweeping tail
represents power.

for the paradox that confronted the Yolngu when they settled
no longer foraged for the starch of the treacherous cycad.
of wheat flour and cane sugar available at the store. It was
be both sweet and safe.

e food

The white wake and the bow wave represent speed. The dorsal fin emphasizes the iron blade of tradition in words, song and ritual. The body represents food. Shark's teeth are used for trimming spears and for *narrtjam*, the shark tooth weapons; all earn their place in the paintings of Dardiwuy, the shark clan.

At the Mission in the early 1970s I admired sets of father-and-son paintings by Sea Snake and Cumulus, which depict *Marrna* the shark. Painting can be a family craft, as Bruegel and Picasso remind us. I bought a painting from each of them. They thrilled me. I kept the father's shark and the son's shark on adjacent barks in the entrance hall of my home. Power, speed, jaws, food, death: what other painting could say as much? The son, Cumulus, was then in his late thirties and worked at the Mission as orderly or policeman, charged with keeping peace and quiet during the nights.

The father, Sea Snake, kept going back with a little band of about 30 people to a remote outstation looking across Captain Flinders' Malay Road to the English Company Islands. In 1976 this little band pulled out, back to the Mission, because they were too beset by sickness, especially in the women, largely of the mental kind. Sea Snake, who has no English, enacted the man with pneumonia in my movie *Aboriginal Healing*. He allowed himself to be therapeutically steamed and smoked by his fellow actors for the demonstration on film. He was rather sick next day, I regret to say; he needed chemotherapy before he mended.

Cumulus seemed to me a flexible

young man, but facing unguessed problems in adaptation. Like others of his generation he has not merely grown up but has grown away from one cultural world and into another. Here is a reminiscence of youth from this young man of the shark totem. The story is of course anglicized—he told it to me in a mixture of dialect and very rudimentary pidgin. I learned crucial lessons from it, including one that he did not intend to teach: that an enthusiasm for fast food of flour and sugar can leave you jaded from satiety, devitalized and corrupted. He knew that something was undermining both him and his family, but he never suspected the new diet. He asked me to put him in my book if it will teach others:

I was born south of Arnhem Bay at Baramburra, on the Gurumaru River flowing into Arnhem Bay. There are two clans in those parts, called Dardiwuy and Naymil. These are in the Dhuwa moiety. When I was growing up, Sea Snake my Bapa taught me the lore of the bush. He made my spear and woomera, and taught me to use them for hunting.

Before I was very old, my Bapa moved to another way in life. He began to spend his time making bark paintings, and selling them to the Mission at Yirrkala. We bought things with the money. We bought clothes and we bought food: sugar, flour, treacle and golden syrup. Now we were always painting for this food. He was always teaching me painting. He taught me the secrets, and I helped him with the paintings. I painted all the time, much more than the other boys. I copied the designs from my Bapa.

I first came out of the bush to Yirrkala Mission when I was six years old. I went to the school for a while, then back in the bush to help my Bapa painting, off and on until I was thirteen. But I was in the bush more than I was at school, so I did not learn to speak much English. We always took plenty of food from the store back to the bush. That was what we ate.

My Bapa taught me how to take colours from stones. Some stones come from the bush, some from the river. Murrngud, the river stone, is pink. The miku stone is red: this is the stone that is everywhere here at this place. Gangul is yellow, from the river in the bush. Black is the junapul if it's a stone, lirriwi if it is burned wood; you call it charcoal. For white we use the clay, gopan, from the cliffs of the big capes.

Mostly I paint on bark. We never paint on the ground as they did in the old days. First of all I find my murrngud, then I cut the stringybark tree with the axe. We always have steel axes in the bush. We flatten the bark with fire and under the sand. We always made our pictures to sell to the Mission, not for the people. The Mission used to buy all of them to sell to Americans for us.

I kept painting our Dardiwuy designs, same as my Bapa. Our river, Wurrululu, is in two parts for the two clans. By order of the leader of the Dardiwuy clan, the shark has to be used in the design. The name of the shark in the Dardiwuy speech is Marrna. Sometimes we drew designs for a hunting story, with Maipunu the turtle, or Dangulji the brolga, or Gunji the jabiru. But mainly we drew the shark ancestor who made the River Wurrululu and then stayed there. Our man ancestor, or god, Djangkawul, made the fresh water shark, the shark in the lagoon. When we paint him, we paint his trail in the water.

I shall briefly interrupt Cumulus to explain the anomaly of freshwater sharks. In the flat mangrove country around Arnhem Bay there are some estuaries opening north towards the bay. In the wet season they overflow their banks to replenish lagoons on either side of the estuary. Some young sharks that have entered these lagoons from the estuary on a high tide are left behind when the water level recedes after the wet season. Now the young sharks become a paradox of nature: sharks in fresh water. Over-feeding in their new habitat upon freshwater food, they sicken. They are easily speared or netted. The flavour of their meat is greatly prized by the clans. The liver in particular, which undergoes expansion, is a delicacy—a pâté, reserved for the elderly and elect. Lagoon sharks are esteemed like the sturgeon of northern waters of the so-called Old World. Cumulus resumed:

At Yirrkala Mission I went to school up to class four. Then I left and came to Elcho Mission with my people, but not to school. This time I was a carpenter, building houses with the missionary for two years. But during the weekends I used to go back to my bark paintings. I took them to Mr Rudder, the teacher in the adult craft centre. So they set me to work full time at the craft centre. I was on a Government Training allowance there, not on piecework. This brought me $17.00 a week, no matter how much I painted.

I can make a small painting in one day, but mostly I do one every week. There were six men there, painting, and we were always painting our own kind of design. Sometimes we carved birds or canoes; or hollow bone poles for the bones of dead relations. Mr Rudder told us what is wanted on the market and we made it. I liked this place because I got a job and was making some money so I made a family near the Mission. I got two wives and five children.

Cumulus talked to me frequently about his father, Sea Snake, and his mothers. Sea Snake has six wives. All had become devoted to the food from the store; even when living away from the Mission back in the bush, they had largely relinquished the quest for bush tucker. Store food was sweet.

Morning Star, the youngest, became 'sick in the head' at their outstation. On one occasion her limbs became stiff and she stared straight ahead without talking and apparently not seeing anybody. It seems it followed

an argument with the Number Four wife. Morning Star was flown from outstation to Mission, and then to hospital in Darwin. After four days Sea Snake came to visit her with a new dress as a present. She was already recovering. Then he gave her $40 which she used to buy more dresses. She is mainly well now, though indolent.

Sea Snake's Number Three wife had to spend a lot of time at East Arm Hospital (for leprosy) in Darwin. Here she had a baby to an Indonesian man. This baby lived only six months; it was taken back to their outstation where it died of malnutrition. Number Three wife next had a baby to a man from Maningrida. By this time she was clearly suffering from severe 'head sickness'. She would sit for weeks doing nothing and crying a lot. Some weeks she was restless and destroyed other people's property. She too requested treatment in Darwin Hospital.

Number Three wife is now mainly well and lives at Cumulus's house at the Mission. Here she looks after two of her children as well as helping with Cumulus's. When she visited her mother and two sisters at Yirrkala, she found that they had 'head sickness' too. She said that all of them must have had head sickness caused by the same curses. While she was at Yirrkala, a middle-aged man took her into his house but after a week or two he said she was no longer welcome there. She keeps well at the house of Cumulus with the aid of a tranquillizing injection (fluphenazine) every three weeks.

What can we make of all this head sickness in these wives? What do they have in common besides their husband? Cumulus resumed his story, explaining his designs, then moved to matters more personal in his own family.

I go to church. Not every Sunday. I don't try to paint Jesus. Bunbaitjun did those Jesus pictures. They are all right on the church wall at Yirrkala, but not on bark. Christ should be on the church wall, Djangkawul on the bark. We call our own designs Grade 1, 2 and 3. Grade 1 is for real sacred designs. At first we tried to stick to the proper sacred ones, but the missionary paid the same for anything, just what is wanted. Now we omit Grade 1 sacred designs; we should be hiding that. So we paint Number 2 designs which is mostly of animals, or Number 3 designs, which is of people, the country, and pretty colours and patterns. We never painted these Number 3 designs in the old days.

A few years ago my two wives became jealous of each other. Then, the younger one desired another man. I saw them with my spirit making eyes at each other. I struck her with a knife. I gashed her with one slice under the shoulder blade. They took me to Darwin. I went to the court. The judge ordered six months, and I went to Fannie Bay Gaol. I worked in the laundry. They cut off two months from the six. I got out on a Saturday and went to the Mission office in Darwin and I was told my seat was already booked on the next plane to the Mission.

When I came back to the Mission I talked to my second wife. She said she was straight with me, though she had been with that man. I took the matter to the village council. Before the meeting, I went down to the Art Centre to see Mr Rudder, and we prayed to Jesus about it together. The council instructed that the man does not come near her any more, and I gave the council my word not to use the knife again. But I didn't mean to do it the first time.

Another time I went to Darwin, for a few weeks. I worked at cutting lawns. I started to drink some alcohol, maybe five cans of beer at a time. But then I worried that if I got drunk, I would kill somebody while I was drunk. Also I worried that other men might kill me while I was drunk. I ended up by not drinking, and taking care of the other Yolngu men who were drinking. I told them that if they got drunk, some other men could come along and hurt them. Then I found out you could not look after drinking men.

Nobody could. So I came home to the Mission. I would not go to Darwin any more, except for a holiday.

This year I got another job as camp orderly on night duty for the Town Council. I go around looking for people breaking the law, like sniffing petrol from cans of coke, or like gambling with cards. One night I took cards to the office five times. Next week the cards were all gone. I used to play the cards before, but not now. My job is Orderly for Cards. From eight o'clock to one o'clock in the morning. About five months ago I caught some boys sniffing petrol, and I took them to the Council. I get $5 a week for this. I just walk around the Yolngu on patrol and watch.

Also I'm a Traffic Orderly. The Town Council says people must ride a motorbike for a year before they have a passenger. I watch for this. If I see they are riding quiet, slow, and by themselves—all right. If they are riding with other Yolngu, or riding too fast, I talk to that riding man. If he is cheeky, I go straight to the Council. If anyone would hit me, I would not hit him back. I would go to the Council.

At the Mission my family get a lot of colds. My father has gone back to the outstation. If people stay out there, and there is no contact with here, there is less colds and flu.

I get so tired from working at night. My head gets sleepy but I can't sleep. Then I go and buy aspirin and cough medicine from the store. This helps my headache. I wear a brown shirt and a policeman's hat when I am on patrol, and I work hard. I get so tired and my head aches so badly. I am a sick man, but I don't know what is wrong with me. I have an enemy, perhaps? Perhaps the card-players curse me?'

What Cumulus omitted to emphasize in his story is how dramatically his diet changed when he and his family left the bush to live from the Mission store. It changed as radically as the diet of those young sharks from the sea who find themselves trapped in the freshwater lagoons. It changed in the direction of the fast food that is sweeping the globe, but a faster food than McDonald's or The Colonel ever envisaged in their wildest dreams.

Here is the standard recipe that I once watched my friend Cumulus prepare at the start of a day. Take a large can with a wire handle. Into it pour one cup of plain flour and two cups of cane sugar. Mix carefully with golden syrup and water until a paste forms. Add salt if desired. Keep the can beside you as you work at your painting, dipping two fingers of the left hand in the paste and sucking them as required.

Most of the Yolngu follow this tin-can recipe. They have no experience of cutlery, crockery or cooking utensils. The tin-can recipe delivers the food. They keep another tin can (locally it is called the billy can) to deliver the tea, which has loads of sugar in it. They do not bother to remove the used tea leaves in the bottom. They drink straight from the can.

I could add to this recipe some prescriptions of my own. Save all the energy you can, for you will have little to spare. Try not to scratch the rash between your fingers as it will bleed easily. Do not rub the cracks at the corner of your mouth. Do not drink your tea too hot as it may hurt your shiny red tongue.

In fieldwork in 1963 I recorded sickness complaints by Carson River clans coming to a dispensary or health centre at Kalumburu, a Spanish mission in the Kimberleys of Australia. This is detailed in a book in preparation.[1] They are tribal people who have given up the nomadic life and the food that nature supplied. They live from choice largely on refined sugar and refined wheat flour from the store.

Why do they choose this kind of food? It is so refined that even the weevils will not touch it. It is cheap and they are poor. It is durable in sealed packets. It is convenient, requiring no culinary effort or kitchens. It is fast and wants no effort to gather. But above all, it is sweet to taste. People who do not find many sweet foods in nature may become 'hooked' when they are exposed to them.

The main medical syndrome at the Spanish mission dispensary was this vague and poorly articulated feeling of ill-health: lassitude, despondency, irritability. These patients asked the nurses at the dispensary simply for 'something to take' as if they perceived that something might go into their mouths to restore well-being and a desire for life. At Kalumburu I called this out-of-sorts complaint 'the dispensary syndrome' and noted that it was most prevalent in the worst-fed people. It was not possible to persuade them that they were eating emptiness. They liked it; it was sweet. We could call it store syndrome.

So the doctors may prescribe 'something to take' while they try to do something about the malnutrition and the infections that people resist so poorly, the dysentery, the hookworm and that constant coughing. But the whole pharmacy, including the psychopharmacy, is of no avail for people who do not have good food.

What is the responsibility of doctors? When it is manifestly impossible to reinstate Primal Therapy comprising two strands: Bush Food Therapy and Bush God Therapy? How does one follow the maxim about putting the stomach first and the brain second? In this case it involves a study of the power of sweet addiction and sweet abuse, before that of anxiety or depression. What doctor can convince a person to go fishing who can get food out of a packet?

These were nature's people who had foraged its garden, like gourmets eating a menu of every conceivable nutrient and taste, always fresh. I have shared 'primal diet' on walks with them. It consists of proteins, fats, vitamins, nutrients, plenty of fibre and plenty of sand. It would keep your teeth strong even if it wears them down. It is the diet to which the human animal is physiologically and metabolically adapted. As a species, humans have eaten it for 99 per cent of their tenure on earth. They departed from it when farming was discovered after the last Ice Age receded and the food glut occurred. A mere 10 000 years before Christ, only yesterday in terms of our occupancy of this dizzily turning planet. Since then, it is humans who have had the dizzy turns.

Physicians often have a habit of filing their correspondence. Here is a painstaking letter I found in my files from Cumulus. It is self-diagnostic when you know his story. And it is sad.

Dear Doctor John,
I got cold or flu. I want you to give me two or four tablets. While we were working at the beaches, I felt sick out there at the beach. I'm feeling sick now. Aches are coming from neck, back, and sides.
Love, Cumulus

This dispensary syndrome, or store syndrome, or saccharine disease, is too vague and ill-defined to classify as pellagra, beri-beri, kwashiorkor, marasmus, scurvy or any other specific nutritional deficiency. It is certainly not equivalent to protein-calorie malnutrition or iron deficiency. Any of these patterns may be seen in it. Australia was particularly at risk because, unlike other advanced countries, it did not have a public health law requiring millers to reinforce the deficiencies of their refined wheat flour. Such a law dramatically reduced deficiency diseases in the United States when it was introduced in the early 1950s; I was studying in the USA shortly after this time and everyone was talking about it. Even the alcoholics under the 'El' in Chicago were suddenly healthier. But Australia, in its wisdom, judged that this public health provision was not needed until very recently, in spite of all my persuasions on behalf of Aborigines.

Since medical students like to be categorical, I tutored on this topic in my hospital under the heading of 'saccharine disease'. The tutorial touched on its many dimensions. The substance abuse most harmful to health in the Western world is arguably not alcohol, or tobacco, or narcotics, or sedatives. It is sugar. In the past hundred years, the per capita consumption of sugar in modern populations increased fourfold. A similar trend applies to cereal foods bulk-manufactured from refined wheat flour. The trend for these foods to increase in popularity must be viewed in the light of epidemiological evidence and animal experiments linking dietary habits with illness. The morbidity of 'saccharine disease' includes obesity and its many ills, dental caries, mature-onset diabetes, high blood pressure, coronary heart disease and lowered resistance to infections.

Most substances which are abused are pleasure reinforcers—alcohol, tobacco, cocaine, opiates, even kava! Sweetness and pleasantness are so closely related that sugar can be classified as an immediate reinforcer. The reinforcement comes from the sweet taste, though some further reinforcement is probably achieved through the calming effect upon limbic centres in the brain from dumping sugar into the bloodstream.

Augmenting the effect of the reinforcement properties is the availability of refined sugar and flour, in contrast with most other foods. Sugar and flour are cheap and durable, easily stored. They are convenient, lending themselves to quick and unceremonious feeding. Little trouble is required to procure and prepare them. As fast foods, they readily become the basis of the eating patterns of individuals who do not have the money, time or kitchen facilities to prepare and eat a broader range of diet. For people today, as for laboratory animals, saccharine disease tends to be related to the schedule for eating, especially to limited culinary effort.

Is saccharine disease (or over-indulgence) an addiction? It fulfils some criteria, though not others. There is no tolerance or dose escalation; there is no withdrawal syndrome—though this is arguable. There is however psychological craving for its immediate reinforcement, sweetness. And there is (as with alcohol, heroin and marijuana) a complex constellation of environmental factors that strengthens the likelihood that substances possessing pleasurable reinforcement will be taken in excess.

The presence of sweet additives in modern food (breakfast cereals, carbonated drinks, sweets, cakes, and breads) enhances their popularity. The advertising and promotion by food vendors of course shapes people's food habits. Sweetness acts as a hidden condiment due to its regular association with protein and other nutrients

present in the modern diet. Saccharine disease has become a substantial threat to individual and public health. It is the scourge of 'Coca-Colonisation'.

While the food industry has established sugar as one of the main components of diet in the West, the effect on the Third World countries which grow the raw material is equally serious. In recent years, roughly half of the eleven million tonnes of sugar consumed annually in the USA is imported from the Dominican Republic, the Philippines and Mexico. A large proportion of arable land in these countries is devoted to the production of sugar, which is exported for foreign exchange that is predominantly spent by the political and economic elites. While the elites may suffer from their engorgement, there is not enough land left over to satisfy the needs of their undernourished local populations.

I would like to share with you a number of reflections on the problems of Cumulus as the Town Orderly. Cumulus is a persevering man, artistically talented, somewhat introspective and solitary. He told us some of the trials of his youth, passing not only through adolescence but through the space voyage between the mesolithic and modern society. It is not just a matter of wrong diet, though I emphasize that lest you should think I discount it.

First, Cumulus and I have problems of communication. He was educated for another world. His art, his painting, served as a bridge between our two worlds. But his lack of the language and technology of the Western world curtails opportunities.

I believe that Cumulus has a problem of temperament. He shows a Yolngu trait which I have called evasion of confrontation. With this trait, tribal men inhibit anger over insults until the hurt cannot be endured and the rage explodes into riots and mayhem. This temperament puts him at a disadvantage in the Western world, which ideally expects irritation to be let out a little at a time. It put him in gaol.

In a polygynous society, Cumulus has a problem over domesticity, just as his father does. Assigned two wives by the kinship system, he finds it is troublesome satisfying both. If he resorts to traditional measures of wife control: move to gaol. Disturbed domesticity at the Mission frequently reveals the old system of polygyny scuffing against the new one of monogamy. Many women in his kinship suffer from head sickness. He does what he can to keep an eye on them. It is demanding for him.

He has a problem over social roles. He is a policeman! This authority figure is unknown in traditional society where the power of religion and medicine is the law. So he endures tension headaches and neurasthenia, while he confiscates the cards from the card games. He treats himself with aspirin from the store.

Cumulus has a real problem over where to send down his roots. Newly conscious of legal deliberations over land rights, traditional Aborigines are dispersing from the settlements in which they congregated after the war in order to raise their flag in little bands in homeland regions. He cannot join his father out there because of his job at the settlement. And he is afraid to live in a big town like Darwin where in theory the opportunities are better. In the big town he becomes tense. He knows very well he cannot use alcohol for reducing his tension. The risk of somebody being killed is too real.

These are some of his problems. Adolescence in Aboriginal people can be a period when happy if not healthy childhood passes into baffled and demoralized adulthood. Cumulus does not blame ill-treatment from whites. Most of the white people he knows have treated him reasonably, courteously, even kindly. He does not complain about them, and he would not complain about them. He does not blame curses.

That is one reason why I have chosen to introduce Cumulus to you. He wants you to know how he feels. In Sydney, European Australians are being told to feel guilty over their genocide of the race. It is stressed by sociologists both white and black, as well as the popular press. I am not sure that guilt is the most effective emotion for arousing vigorous and helpful effort from the European side. Interest and challenge may be. Guilt brings a painful ambivalence. I have seen Australian doctors, my colleagues, sensitive to the anger expressed to them by young radical Aborigines, turn away from them. This is no time to turn away from youth, above all from Aboriginal youth.

Our new indigenous townships have a dilemma of how far to assist their youth stay afloat, how far to let them sink or swim by themselves. That is the behavioural health problem for a people who have yet to develop their behavioural health system. Few doctors are coming forward to make their career in this too challenging speciality. We train specialists for city dwellers. In consequence we fail to train doctors for these harassed detribalizing people who try to run their own behavioural health system.

To return to Cumulus. I find a

fable in the misadventure of the young shark, which is enshrined in my mythic paintings by Sea Snake and Cumulus.[2] This shark swam out of the clear air and wide seas to become trapped in the land-locked lagoon. The teeming life in fresh water made him sick but he had to stay in it.

Is it the lagoon shark of whom we speak, or is it Cumulus? His story is an opportunity to appreciate him in this new environment. That is our invitation: to know him, in his new context.

If we really know him, something may follow. His is not an exotic disease, like this shark in the lagoon; he is a deserving and talented man with difficulties, who can be helped, for a start, by a proper diet. Oh, the treachery of white food!

1   Cawte J (in preparation) *The Mind of Early Man: Psychology in Ancient Australia.*

2   Now donated to the University of New South Wales. Cumulus, Sea Snake and the other artists have been informed of this.

TREACHERY OF WHITE FOOD

I ceased work at the clinic before fou
My head felt too thick to write up th
myself I would do it that evening. T
stepped out onto the dirt road that s
and vacant bay.

by the fir

IN

The Health Centre at the Mission on Elcho Island is called Njalkanbuy (at least it is called that on its stationery), which means 'eagle's nest'. The letterhead has a drawing of a disgruntled eagle apparently perched on a termite's castle. Yolngu are ever poetic. This does not imply that there is any eagle's nest hereabouts, merely that there is a soaring outlook having a panoramic view over the bay to a small island in middle distance.

Beyond the horizon towards the declining sun lies the old parent Mission, the first founded in these parts, Milingimbi. It is sited in the Crocodile Islands. I wandered down the path to the edge of the cliff, wishing I had the wings of an eagle to find a cool current of air to rest upon for a while.

ock on that afternoon. There were no more patients.

se sheets with the proper brevity and clarity; I promised

eat was oppressive and I felt enervated and groggy. I

ed down to the top of the cliff overlooking that vast

st
TENTION

The tide was out, far out. On the edge of the exposed reef I espied Billy Reid, fishing, while the surf slapped at the rocks at his feet. From this distance Billy looked small and lonely, like a child, although he is of large stature. His head was shaded by a wide cowboy hat. Billy is a Kamileroi, an Aboriginal man of Emu descent, who hails from Bourke on the Darling River in the northern plains of New South Wales. The central part of his tribe was the 'Pilliga Scrub mob', he tells us. An artist, he illustrated the journal that I produced for Aboriginal health workers.[1] He sometimes came with me on trips to far places. But Billy found it perplexing to mix with the Aboriginal people on this island, and they with him. Islander and inlander people are poles apart in outlook. So he was often on his own, line in hand, engaged at his favourite pastime.

I looked about for my daughter Alice who had gone down there with him: she was probably attacking rock oysters somewhere with a hammer. Was she wearing a hat? I wondered. She is red-headed and should respect the sun up here, but it is not always easy to persuade young women to dress for the elements.

I clambered down that precipitous trail on the face of the cliff to pass the time with Billy. As I was approaching he appeared to cast out his line too strongly; it missed its aim on the sandy bottom, and the hook became snagged in the coral reef.

'Damn!' said Billy to me, to the gulls, to the littoral at large. 'There goes my second line, and I'm short of gear. No fish for dinner tonight!'

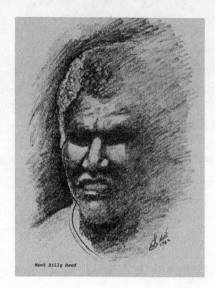

Meet Billy Reed

I mentally weighed the chances of recovering the hook and line, and the wisdom of trying. It was snagged in shallow water only a few feet below the surface. The surf today would keep the stingers elsewhere, so the water seemed safe. The bottom was sandy and you could see the rocks well enough to avoid them. I did not expect Billy to go in after it; he copes with a childhood injury to his foot which would make that difficult. I took off my shoes and pants and left them with my wrist watch in Billy's care as I told him to keep the nylon line taut. I used the line to steady myself as I waded into the water and levered my way cautiously towards that small patch of coral reef, which looked no bigger than the floor of an average room of an average house. It was easy to find the place with that taut line to guide me to it. Gingerly I groped for the hook, standing unsteadily, waist high in the surging water that was frothing over that small reef. At length the hook and sinker came free, and Billy started to reel in the line.

This undid me! Instantly I lost my anchor, my point of reference. Losing my balance, I slipped and fell, lacerating the ball of my left foot on some jagged coral. An ordinary accident, but an extraordinary pain! It was as if a stingray had attacked me with its lightning strike. I could do no more than float off this reef to the sandy bottom, and crawl my way out of the sea, blood streaming behind me. I thought of alerting Billy to my predicament, but he is moderately deaf and would not have heard me over the splashing of the surf.

Once out of the water I held Billy's shoulder to examine the laceration. It was about as long as my little finger: deep, jagged, with a small artery spurting blood in the base. I tied my handkerchief tightly around the foot; then I replaced my sock and my shoe with difficulty. With Billy's help I somehow hobbled painfully up the cliff path, making my way to the top and to Eagle's Nest.

It would mean calling back the nurse to dress my laceration. I was mentally debating whether to have her suture it or strap it strongly enough to hold it together. I knew that suturing was normally preferable, but I had in my mind a memory of a football match which the ratings of a naval ship, a destroyer, had played on a patch of ground mixed with fragmented pieces of coral, near Honiara in the Solomon Islands. I was then the ship's surgeon. I had not watched those boys play their football, though I was aware of the keg of beer that they had standing in the shade to treat their dehydration. None of the abrasions that those boys sustained healed properly, by the first intention: they exuded green pus for weeks, as their defence system tried to handle minute coral fragments embedded in the flesh, not to mention any algae that infested the coral fragments. That cruise in the Pacific became a nightmare for those naval ratings and their surgeon alike. I wondered if I should be destined for a like fate, if my laceration had chanced to pick up some coral pieces within its torn tissue. If that proved to be the case, it might be better not to suture it in the usual way, but to let it drain, to heal 'by the second intention'. The slow and painful way.

On arriving at the clinic I found not the nurse but one of the Yolngu health workers waiting for me in a state of some agitation. The motor of his vehicle was still running. He wanted me to come, this instant, to see a disturbed man who he said had gone mad and was threatening his family with an axe. It seemed that my own minor surgery would have to wait its turn.

We climbed aboard his vehicle and drove down the hill to this man's rabbit hutch of an iron cottage. The fellow would not come outside; he was too afraid. Inside, we found him perched up on the stove like a trapped bird, his relatives marshalled on the floor around it. He had an axe at his side. There were no chairs or any other furniture in that inferno of a kitchen. A doctor has an advantage with psychotics and people in panic: a doctor can generally make the medical role clear, and is usually outside the system of persecutions that are driving such persons to take these desperate measures.

We talked, and I got the story. He had been cursed. He was hearing threatening spirits in the air around

him, and he even thought he had a lizard in his guts. We talked some more, enough to get him to agree to take a tablet from a bottle I had brought. I told him that it should make the spirits leave. He swallowed that tablet, and I promised him that the lizard might stop chewing on his bowels. He agreed to see me first thing in the morning after the sleep I promised. The health worker borrowed his axe before we left—he had a job for it to do at home, he said. It was not needed here any more.

By the time I returned to my own quarters any thought of organizing sutures for my laceration had receded. I washed it in the sink with soap and water. The bleeding had stopped. I bound it with a dry adhesive bandage—it was a new kind of bandage, an improvement over the kind I used when I was last a casualty officer. At that time we sewed up people's wounds with horse hair. It was not easy to tie knots with horse hair . . . I was weary and slept. I believe that the cursed man whom I had just seen also slept, before he hurt someone during his attack of schizophrenia.

Next morning my daughter Alice and I were equally casualties; she was in more distress than I. She had an allergic reaction to sandfly bites that a chance swarm inflicted on her the previous day on the beach. Sandflies do not fly like flies or mosquitoes: they just jump out at you in a battalion if you disturb them. Alice had no immunity to the pests, like the local people. Her lesions were ugly, not bites now but weals and blebs, all around her legs. She was very sick with it, so I took her to the clinic to see Sister Anna, who knew just what to do. She gave her a dose of antihistamine, a warning about clothing protection against sandflies, and an application of Kater's and Calamine Lotion, a Northern Territory Health Department preparation. She gave her the remains of the ten-ounce bottle to take home.

I was debating whether to seek Sister Anna's help for the laceration of my left foot. It was giving me a good deal of pain and, in a bizarrely inappropriate way for a doctor, I had almost persuaded myself during the night that this pain was good for me. I lived a life free of pain, most of the time, and I had forgotten its blessings. Being in pain intensifies your appreciation of life, and your gratitude for your health! It offers you the satisfaction of summoning your stoicism and withholding your complaints. Pain, if not too prolonged, is a moral reminder, a kind of bliss. But then I decided that this Puritan ethic was reckless, and I showed her my foot. She bade me lie on my back on the surgery table while she examined it. She cleaned it up in a kidney bowl. She instilled a generous amount of Neotracin powder—she told me it was soluble and would absorb. Then she sutured it. She applied a much better dressing than the one I had.

While she was doing all this I could not see the sole of my own foot, so I watched Anna's face. Suddenly I perceived what a beautiful woman she was. It hit me. She was not simply what a nurse should be: practical, skilled, cool, efficient, even kind. There was something blessed here. She wore a detached air of divinity. What beauty a nurse can assume for a man in pain! She was beautiful. While she worked she glanced at my face. Where is any author in the world who teaches such beauty as a woman's eye? Her glance was serious, significant, imparting serenity.

CHAPTER THIRTEEN

'You must get a lot of satisfaction out of nursing procedures well done,' I said.

'None,' she replied.

'None?' I was startled to hear it.

'None at all. I take procedures as a matter of course. It goes without saying you must do them properly. I get my satisfaction from people. I'm more interested in counselling. When I leave here, I think I'll join a downtown Mission clinic in Sydney—a place where they care for adolescent drug addicts. I'd like to assist these kids, talk with them, offer them some other way, encourage them. These people up here don't need my help so much.'

She changed the subject, bringing up the epilepsy of a staff member: she was dissatisfied with his medication and wanted to discuss a possible change. I advised her as best I could.

How the Yolngu must have loved this Sister Anna! How disappointed they would be to hear that she planned to leave them. She was efficient, serene, courteous. I felt I loved her, like them. My laceration healed by the first intention. I dressed it each night. The pain soon left, but I hobbled around with a stick for a month or two. That coral wound spared me its more sinister impositions. Anna had judged correctly in suturing yesterday's wound. I thanked her in my heart. Her action was blessed.

There is a high rate of lacerations in the Yolngu, particularly of the feet, as they go unshod over rough terrain. Healing is often slow because of the poor hygiene and worse nutrition. Healing is unreliable; the one thing that you can rely on is complications occurring. Wounds heal by the 'second intention'. The Yolngu apply their own remedies which can bring on a few complications. They say that urinating on an open wound hardens it and removes the pus. They apply all kinds of gum and sap from plants and trees. They say that maggots in the base of a wound eat the dead meat and soak up the pus, making it clean. So they do not mind blowflies, and they do not oppose their maggots. I will settle for Hagedorn needle sutures, Neotracin dusting power, Hansaplast patent dressings if sutures are not possible, and the attention of a prompt and confident nurse, with the glance of Sister Anna.

There is a medico-political movement at some of these remote townships to displace nurses by health workers 'who belong to the people'. I hope that nurses and health workers will always be in close partnership at these places. I would not care to see one group work without the other. The health worker needs the rigour of the nurse. The nurse needs the culture of the health worker. I never saw a nurse who knew much about cursing, though cursing is the set of ideas which determines the response the patient makes in many cases. The nurse usually does not want to bother about it, any more than the visiting doctor does. So they label the patient's unexpected response to what should be obvious treatment, as 'low compliance'. This is one reason I have penned these recollections.

But the chief hazard highlighted in these pages is not the everyday malice between humans so much as the havoc inflicted by the ecology. Aboriginal people in settlements are martyrs to the ecology of Australia. Until and unless that can be relieved, health and welfare will not change significantly.

Talking with Anna, it did not take me long to discover that she was a devout Christian, which motivated her

to undertake her unusual and difficult work. She discussed with me how her Christian ethic shaped her work in this community, and would shape it in the city when she quit. Her ethic led her to make a visiting list of deserving cases and to walk to their places of residence. Deserving cases on her list are the neglected children—some of them are exceptional children, she was sure. They are the neglected old folk. They are the handicapped—the blind, the deaf, the crippled, the backward. They are the drug and alcohol abusers. They are the inadequate, and those who can't cope for want of a job or a budget. They are the headache complainers—I told Anna that up here, people who complain insistently of headaches are often saying that they are depressed in some way. They never say 'depressed'. They are the people who hear imaginary spirits. Much of that can be alleviated by our attention.

A lot of sufferers out there! Anna had them on her visiting list. I was glad that her Christian ethic encompassed them all. It was heartening to find a young Christian who was working out her own way to do it. She seemed uninterested in promoting the doctrine of salvation through Jesus Christ or threats of damnation in hell. No rhetoric about the Holy Ghost. This gave new heart to a sloppy agnostic like myself, beginning to feel out of date in the New Wave of fundamentalist missionaries. I do not know where Sister Anna has gone, but the scar on my foot that healed 'by the first intention' sometimes brings back this small miracle with gratitude. God bless her.

1 Reid W (1982) *Billy Reid's Sore Skins. For Aboriginal Health Workers and Others.* Text by Brien Walder and Danny Beran. University of Queensland Printery.

In chapter 1, I used the term 'pulse' f
Aboriginal settlements, I felt that th
Balanda. Nobody on Elcho Island w
cups. But mostly the pulse is strong a
eyes in the pages of this book.

A NEW *pulse* ARN

Two features of the pulse particularly strike the medical person. The first is the refusal—so far—of Galiwin'ku to yield to drink. There's a level of sobriety that fosters health, progress and harmony. Rarely is a visiting doctor called to deal with injuries inflicted by drunks. In other communities where I have offered my services, it is common to see good folk become so plastered as to fight and brawl violently.

The other miracle at Galiwin'ku—for a doctor—is the baby boom. These Yolngu are no dying race; they are expanding as fast as humanity can. Every hundred people (man, woman and child) bring forth each year up to six new babies, healthy enough to

ie throb of life or vitality in Galiwin'ku. Of the many
ie showed a promising partnership between Yolngu and
laim that their pulse beats serenely. Naturally, there are hic-
resilient, even to the exotic threats that have opened our

in
HEM LAND

thrive. Anxious watchers say that the birthrate is too high for the good of the family, and the children themselves. We have to look at that.

How was this achieved? As I look back to the dawn of Galiwin'ku I think of the notable contributors: some outstanding Yolngu leaders and the earliest Methodist missionaries.

The Yolngu leaders who facilitated the establishment of the colony at Galiwin'ku were indeed outstanding. They could be called statesmen, men of peace, bearers of the olive branch. They persuaded the Yolngu clans to live together. It was frightening for Yolngu to live side by side with other clans who may have been traditional

foes, smarting under grievances from feuds still active in memory.

Peace between the clans! Galiwin'ku brought the blessing of harmony, where tension and mistrust had always ruled. Before long, the new town attracted the large Galpu clan whose territory lay to the east, near the Gulf of Carpentaria, where the Mission stands at Yirrkala. Galpu felt threatened by their longstanding dispute with the powerful Riratjingu owners of that region, so they emigrated to the new haven of Galiwin'ku even though they were then outsiders, beyond the pale.

A leader of this pacification process at Galiwin'ku was Badangga, of the Wongurri clan. I was never to meet him; he died before my arrival. I saw what he had left. One outcome of his politics is discussed by Professor Ronald Berndt in *An Adjustment Movement in Arnhem Land*.[1]

A number of clan leaders, led by Badangga,[2] had made an unprecedented departure from custom. They brought out their sacred carved idols, like burial poles, representing ancestors, from their hiding places, and displayed them openly in the middle of Galiwin'ku, just beside the stream. They had chosen to deprive these idols of their mystery and power over life and death, now that the clans had to live amicably together. The women, suddenly seeing these unviewable, unutterable objects for the first time, fled into the bush for safety, fearing that they would die. Some stayed away for weeks before hearing that it was safe to return. Today, this set of idols still stands by the Galiwin'ku stream, and are called 'The Memorial'. The idols are unpainted, neglected, rotting in the rain and fading in the sun. Nobody pays the slightest respect to them.

Two other leaders who helped to strengthen the pulse of the new village were Wili Walalipa, of Macassan descent, and David Burrumarra, a brilliant individual who picked up English so quickly that he became the first Yolngu schoolteacher. The influence of each man cannot be overestimated. Wili showed a more cosmopolitan outlook than most of his companions, perhaps because of his Macassan derivation. As well, his appearance was different. He and I talked about what the Macassans had brought; Wili had in fact travelled overseas with them, I think to Singapore. His English was hard to follow because of its accent, but somehow his presence modified the indivisibility of the Yolngu, calling Macassar to mind.

David Burrumarra has been well commemorated. He proclaimed me his clan brother shortly after my arrival, and took much time to teach me the beliefs and history of his clan, the Warramirri. It was on my arrival in the seventh year of my visits that he and his 'committee' were waiting for me at the airstrip, and told me that they had decided to have me write a book about them. I promised that they would receive any royalties.

When in 1993 *The Universe of the Warramirri* was finally published, six participants came down from Arnhem Land to Sydney for its launching, escorting the ageing Burrumarra, who was now blind from cataracts. The University of New South Wales lodged the group at New College, perhaps because I had donated my beautiful collection of bark paintings from Galiwin'ku to the university. When the escort went home, I admitted Burrumarra to the Prince of Wales Hospital in Randwick. When eye surgery had previously been contemplated at Casuarina Hospital in Darwin, his family had been warned that an anaesthetic posed risks for his heart, so they had taken him home. Under my care in Sydney, he opted for the surgery without general anaesthetic. All went well; the eye surgeon, Dr Geoff Cohn, speedily extracted the cataracts on successive days while I held my brother's hands under the sterile sheet and soothed him. It was not hypnosis; he just trusted and co-operated Rrapu, his daughter, then took him home to a big feast. He saw pretty well for the rest of his life.

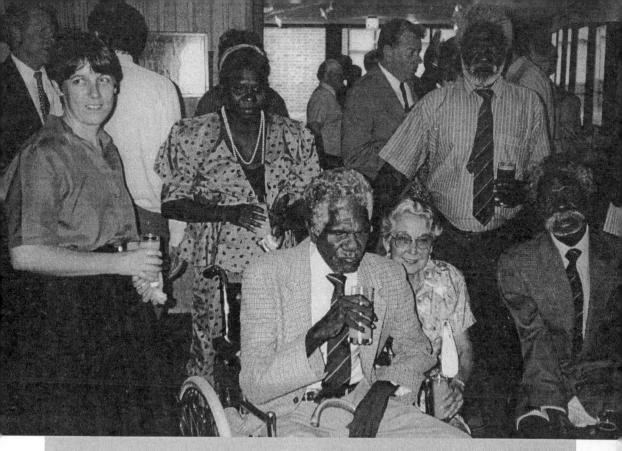

David Burrumarra (seated centre) surrounded by friends and relations at the launch of the book he instigated, *The Universe of the Warramirri*, in January 1994 at the University of New South Wales. Professor John Niland, Vice-Chancellor, is also present (far rear left) and the author Professor John Cawte (rear centre).

Burrumarra also formed a friendship with a teacher at Shepherdson College, Ian MacIntosh, which in 1994 resulted in an informative book, *The Whale and the Cross: Conversations with David Burrumarra*, full of historic photographs of early Galiwin'ku. One shot depicts a proud Burrumarra seated before a Remington typewriter. MacIntosh's title is well chosen to represent the two religions of this leader: his own totemism and Christianity. He seemed a man who craved the 'cargo' of the white man and who, because of this, had to live with some ambivalence in his own personality, and to endure the ambivalence he aroused in his own people.

Within the gathered clans, clan leaders could not retain their tradi-

tional place. Capable young men were coming along who had been learning from the missionaries, in the trades, in the English language, in Western ideas, and in the Christian religion. They came to the fore. I formed a closeness with George Danygambul. It grew stronger when I could help him medically for his bronchitis, a widespread complaint in this village. Eventually, I had to give my opinion that breathing would not get any better while he continued to smoke. George accepted this advice and gave up smoking. Not only did he accomplish this feat, but he formed a group of six other men who also gave up the weed. He will not think that my telling this tale is any breach of his privacy; he himself has already told the story in an issue of the little journal I founded, *The Aboriginal Health Worker*. On my last visit to Galiwin'ku we were delighted to meet again. He was in fine health, holding the appointment of chairman of management of the outlying communities. It was a most convivial reunion.

Smoking to excess is a constant problem in Aboriginal communities, as it is elsewhere. I detected a number of individuals whose chest signs suggested that they might be suffering from lung cancer, probably too advanced to treat. The experience sent my mind back to my days in medical school in the 1940s. The connection between smoking and lung cancer was not established, and various causes were sought. Our Professor of Pathology, J B Cleland (later Sir John)[3] told us that he had been required to conduct autopsies on more than one hundred Aborigines and had not found lung cancer in any of them. Why were they spared? It made him wonder—could the tar roads universal in the cities but rare in tribal areas be a cause? He also observed that many of them liked to chew rather than smoke tobacco. Learning this, I packed sticks of Sunlight plug tobacco to take as gifts for helpers, on my early trips. But chewing was not in vogue in Arnhem Land! The Yolngu sat in a ring, inhaling suffocating quantities of smoke from a Macassan pipe; several of the lung cancer victims followed this habit. The women more commonly smoked from crabs' claws.

George Danygambul became one of the community-appointed chairmen of the Town Council that took over administration of the village. He was followed by a sequence of capable

chairmen, who brought stability and rationality to public matters. One of the Galiwin'ku regulations was that alcohol be banned on the island. They well understood that anxiety is high in individuals trying to adapt to Western life, so that many will look to drink for relief. But drink is addicting; after a period, drinkers become too shaky to stop. Then prudence vanishes and frustration and violence take over.

Of course, prohibition rules can be flouted by those who fly in from the big town with 'grog' concealed in their baggage. The rule cannot be policed, as America attempted in the era of bootleggers and speakeasies. But the Council regulation abides: it confers benefit on all those anxious souls who are readily addicted—possibly a majority, in my estimate. When Yolngu go away to towns like Darwin or Nhulunbuy, they often become 'plastered'. Partly it's the company they keep, but it's also the phobia that afflicts Aboriginal people when they leave home for strange places.

While I hasten to compliment the Galiwin'ku chairmen and their councils on their objectives and capability, there have been failures in communication between us. Not infrequently these failures have been my fault. The occasion that I remember best concerns my invitation to three Arnhem Landers to accompany me as delegates to a conference in Ujung Pandang, the former city of Macassar, in South Sulawesi, formerly Celebes. I included a female health worker in my group. The Chairman of Council became hurt that I omitted to consult him over the choice of delegates. I explained to him that I was not using the government's money. It was my own. That was hardly satisfactory; he should have been consulted. I could only apologise for my oversight.

The earliest Methodist missionaries were led by Harold Shepherdson. Their contribution to the success of this venture was deeply humane and compassionate. It became remarkably diverse in its scope. Apart from preaching the Christian faith and promoting values associated with Methodism, it provided teaching in basic trades, education of children in school and provision of nursing and public health. Behind this broad program was the aim to hand over these responsibilities to the Yolngu, as soon as they were able to accept them. Let us look separately at some of these strands of missionary work.

I am not the right person to comment on the value of Christian preaching, contrasted with the traditional worship of animal species, basic to Yolngu totemic belief. Different religions spar with each other. I well recall the aside uttered to me by Burrumarra, as we left the church one hot Sunday morning, after an endless service:

> God the father,
> God the Son,
> God the Holy Ghost,
> Laintjun, Djankawul, Wawilak.
> Mix them all up
> and make a big mountain of bother.

He could have been summarizing the history of human strife, not only holy wars.

Teaching in the school—later to be named Shepherdson College—was essential but, like so many other Mission services, difficult to evaluate. So much depended on the individual. Some pupils advanced rapidly, but in the whole town the use of English remained, and remains, low. Clan lan-

guages are spoken, although the school selected Gupapuyngu as a 'lingua franca'. Those who speak English do so as a second language. Introspective individuals may speak no English. The English that is spoken is reserved to a restricted range of contexts. It fails in others. Michael Cook, an interpreter in English and Jambapuyngu, recently gave us a revealing study[4] of miscommunication in the courtroom; it is based upon a coroner's case that examined the killing of a poor psychotic Yolngu who was shot while Task Force police were apprehending him on the island.

The people's limited use of English was one reason I visited Galiwin'ku twice a year for over 20 years. I had to learn what I could of the vernacular to communicate with them, and to let them communicate with me. This two-way talk is essential to the practice of my calling—if one is to learn anything of the personalities.

Finally, we must come to the mission nurses. Upon them depended so much of the health and security that marked the Galiwin'ku community—and the population boom that surprised me. Boom? One should perhaps call it an explosion. It certainly calls for comment.

Some of these young Mission nurses seemed to me outstanding examples of womanhood—though a few have been men, like Hilton Jones. Many might call them the true healers of Arnhem Land. They are highly trained and self-sacrificing. In my earlier years at Galiwin'ku, when there were fewer nurses, I helped them more directly and was closely consulted. Later, as their forces grew, I was less in demand; I still found them invaluable shapers of community life.

The Mission nurse's work was by

no means confined to the sick bay, a building relocated several times during my years, from the beach to the foot of the cliff and, finally, to the majestic place called Njalkanbuy (Eagle's Nest) that overlooks the vast Castlereagh Bight. Some nurses presided over the sick bay; others moved into the community, attending to people who failed to come to the clinic, and to public health issues, such as health and nutrition. One—how well I recall Sister Ros Brand!—focused on pets; at my request she even wrote an article, 'Caring for Your Dog' in the June 1979 issue of *The Aboriginal Health Worker*. Do nurses stay longer at missions than at government settlements? One commonly heard this! If true, it could account for closer contact and deeper intimacy at the former. The same would apply to teachers and tradesmen. Aboriginal people often said that they had faith in people who came back after their first vacation—and kept coming back! Did missions have that merit?

One of the many challenges for nurses of Aboriginal people is to reinforce the place of Aboriginal health workers and to encourage this vocation. Nurses see the health worker's task as being one of communication, with supervision of health behaviours and promoting understanding of what matters in health. Clinical procedures are not at the core of it. How much responsibility should health workers take? Should they be taught to dress wounds, and to deliver babies? Such procedures form the accepted duties and ethics of the nursing profession. I was only too happy to let the two parties work out the division of duties. No rules could be applied in such situations; some nurses are inherently democratic, and some authoritarian.

The population boom that turned Galiwin'ku from a village of 350 into a town of over 1500 (still growing) during my years of attendance can in part be attributed to the nurses. Improved regular nutrition is a factor that determines a woman's fertility. Interruption to the female diet can reduce fertility.[5] There is little doubt that nurses improved the level of nutrition, especially among the young women. As well, girls now reached puberty early, when most of them were obliged to subscribe to the marriage assignments made at the time of their birth. The Mission steadfastly declined to influence the traditional marriage arrangements, characterised by polygyny, multiple wives, and the 'promise' of baby girls to future husbands, leaving the girls no choice. Most girls go to their assigned husbands at puberty. All this increases the rate of population growth.

The Mission nurses offered the modern methods of family planning to young women, including the pill. Acceptance was low. Nurses told me that husbands were keen to have all the children they could. It paid off financially, when there were few other sources of income. Most young mothers were eligible for two pensions from the government: one for unmarried mothers (those not 'officially' married) and one as an unemployment benefit.

With improved antenatal and postnatal care, most of the babies survived; 'failure to thrive' in young children came later on, especially in the wake of hookworm, anaemia, multiple infections and unbalanced nutrition. Nurses privately vented the fear that there were now too many young children, with too few parents to care for them. The reality also included the settled lifestyle: now that families had abandoned the nomadic life, there was less for mothers to teach their children about the ways to survive.

Some nurses—and some teachers—blamed the growing imbalance between parents and children for disciplinary problems at school, including under-attendance. During this period, the habit of sniffing petrol became widespread. Gangs of children would wander about, holding a coke can of petrol under their shirts, sniffing it to the point of excitement or collapse. Drivers did their best to lock away supplies of petrol, but never successfully. When kids want drugs, they usually get them. A further concern about 'sniffing' was the damage that lead poisoning from petrol can cause in the brain, with slowed mental functioning and epilepsy, as well as delinquency and delirium.

The nurses' day was accordingly a mix of satisfaction and frustrations. But that is the way of life at Galiwin'ku; and probably at most Aboriginal communities in the country. A unique feature of Galiwin'ku is the proportion of helpers, white and dark, who talk about these problems and look for the means of

healing. Healing is displacing magic as the foundation of healthy living. This is no task for the faint-hearted. At Galiwin'ku, Yolngu leaders and mission staff—at least in its early days—joined forces in the challenge to overcome the ideological shock that confronts all Aboriginal communities. 'Healing' is the outcome of united effort.

We may come to the conclusion that on Elcho Island, in the Reserve of Northeast Arnhem Land, massive stresses and problems are indeed looming, but they are being tackled by a collaborative partnership of black and white. Credit is due to both races: may its pulse continue beating in this way.

1 Berndt R (1962) *An Adjustment Movement in Arnhem Land* Mouton, Paris.

2 The name Badangga is of Macassan origin. It comes from 'deng' for 'boat captain'.

3 'Burtie' Cleland was also a prominent botanist. There are more species of native plants named after his discovery (*clelandii*) than for any other investigator.

4 Cook M 'Aboriginal evidence in the cross-cultural courtroom' In Diana Eades (ed) (1995) Language in Evidence University of New South Wales Press.

5 Laughlin C D and Brady I A (eds) (1978) *Extinction and Survival in Human Populations* Columbia University Press New York.

Since this book is written for the general reader, unusual or vernacular words have been kept to a minimum. A few are explained here that may be of special interest. A more extensive glossary may be found in *The Universe of the Warramirri* (1993).

Arafura
The sea lying between Arnhem Land in the south and Irian Jaya in the north. The origin of the name is obscure; it is neither Aboriginal nor Portuguese. It may derive from the Latin word aurifera (gold-bearing) found on the charts of early navigators.

Arnhem
Arnhem Land was named by the crew of the Dutch ship Arnhem, which came to Cape Arnhem and Arnhem Bay in 1623. The ship itself received its name from the city of Arnhem in Holland.

Balanda
White man, from the Macassan 'Hollander', a Dutchman.

Bapi
Generic name for snake. Pythons of swamp or rocks (Witiji, Gunthurra) are Dhuwa. Venomous snakes of the bush (Ludhay) are Yirritja. The rainbow serpent, hero of the monsoon season (Julunggul) is Dhuwa.

Bilimbirr
A healing well, dug in the sand like a trench, for the ritual revitalisation of those suffering from fatigue, weakness or depression.

Borrpoi
Deadliness and black magic, corresponding to puri-puri in Papua New Guinea. Items belonging to the target of malice are stolen and roasted to bring pain and redness to the corresponding part by sympathetic magic. Examples of borrpoi, quoted in the chapter 'Intent to inflame' relate to clothing, saliva and imprints on the ground. Also means payback and leprosy.

Bunggul
A general term for ceremonies, camp or secret. The bunggul following death may be the most elaborate, circumcision the next. A marriage is given little, if any, bunggul.

Buralgor
The land of dead souls for the Dhuwa moiety. Also spelled Bralku.

Dhuwa
One of the two halves, or intermarrying moieties, of society.

Dirrimu
Man

Djankawul
The hero who founded the Dhuwa clans came by canoe from the island called Buralgor to the present Port Bradshaw coastline, with his two sisters. They journeyed through the country, creating the waterholes. Djankawul stole the sacred totems of the women, which placed them in the subservient role they have had ever since. Also spelled Djanggawul. (For his story, see Louis A Allen, *Time Before Morning: Art and Myth of the Australian Aborigines*.

Djarada
A love song, surreptitiously voiced with intent to make the admired one yield.

Galka
Sorcery or magical killer. Raggalk is an alternative form in some dialects.

Gaywarr
Deadly sea wasp; the killing jellyfish.

Gunampi
Vernacular name for ciguatera fish poisoning.

Gurindin
Pidgin for 'quarantine' located on Channel Island near Darwin for the care of infectious patients suffering Hansen's disease.

Kunapipi
In Yolngu mythology, Kunapipi is a man-eater and a central figure in the Kunapipi fertility and initiation rituals. The fertility mother gave birth to all the first children. Also spelled Gunabibi.

Laintjun
The hero who founded the Yirritja clans. He came from the waves of Blue Mud Bay during parching drought and famine. He showed the Yolngu how to make fish traps in the swamps, and taught the use of fire for hunting, cooking and pleasure. He gave each clan a language and a territory, and taught the rules for gifts and marriage. (For his story, see John Cawte, *The Universe of the Warramirri*.)

Macassar
Seaport in the Celebes whence fleets of praus set forth to collect trepang, pearlshell and pearls from the coast of Arnhem Land. Now named Ujung Pandang in South Sulawesi. Also spelled Makasar.

Makarata
Ritual bloodletting, by a spear thrust through a submissive thigh, to settle an old score.

Mala
Clan. As among, for example, the Scots, Yolngu are divisible into groups of families which claim descent from a common ancestor. These lineages have interests in common, such as territory, the regulation of marriage and rituals. Languages are related among adjacent clans.

Manymak
Excellent, very good indeed. Often a term of approval or agreement in conversation. Pronounced 'Mainmark'.

Marayin
Ceremonial of the creative epoch, or the pantheon of ancestral heroes, whose mysteries are concealed. Corresponds to the 'Dreamtime' of Central Australian tribes. Also Maraian.

Marngit
Wise man; sage; healer of ills; medicine man. Also Marngitj in related dialects.

Merringor
Clan warfare. Some clans have been wiped out by this, within living memory of the Yolngu. Sometimes spelled Maringo.

Mielk
Woman

Mintji
Funeral, mortuary.

Moiety
One of the two intermarrying units into which a tribe is divided on the basis of unilateral descent. For the Yolngu the moieties are called Yirritja and Dhuwa. (Moiety is from Latin medietas, meaning 'half'.)

Narra
Private ceremony for men alone.

Nanidji
Alcohol, liquor of any kind.

Ngata
Food, of any kind.

Puri puri
The name in Papua New Guinea for black magic or sorcery. Corresponds to the Yolngu term Borrpoi.

Raggalk
Sorcerer or magical killer. Alternative form of Galka.

Rangga
Carved idols of ancestors usually kept secret, brought out for sacred ceremonies. Part of the Marayin.

Reri
Sickness

Rom
Traditional body of law. Includes: marriage forbidden within clan or moiety; women punished for spying on Marayin, the secret objects; promising of baby girls for future marriage; avoidance rules for near relatives; polygyny.

Trepang
Malay word for the sea cucumber (Holothuria edulis), prolific in shallow seas off Arnhem Land. Not harvested by Yolngu because it is poisonous. Boiling removes the poison. Dried and exported to China, it becomes a popular food with rejuvenating properties, called by them sea-ginseng. Also named beche-de-mer and sea slug.

Wawalag
Also spelled Wawilak. See Burrumarra's quote on p. 133. In Yolngu mythology, the two Wawalag sisters outraged the Rainbow Snake Julunggul (Yurlunggur) by profaning the sacred well with menstrual blood. The Snake swallowed the sisters, their babies and their bitch dogs. He was boasting of his meal when an ant bit him, making him vomit them all up again. .

Wongarr
Creation; akin to God in the Old Testament; maker.

Yirritja
one of the two halves, or intermarrying moieties, of society.

Yolngu
The Aboriginal people of northeast Arnhem Land. Called 'Murngin' by W L Warner in A Black Civilisation.